Child and Adolescent Obesity

Child and Adolescent Obesity

A Practical Approach to Clinical Weight Management

Edited by

Dr Laura Stewart
*Lead Consultant, Appletree Lifestyle
Consultancy, Scotland, UK*

WILEY Blackwell

Contents

5 Changing Behaviours 89
Laura Stewart

6 Physical Activity, Screen Time and Sleep 105
Laura Stewart

Child Obesity – Foreword

When Dr Stewart (Laura) asked me to write the foreword for her book, it immediately triggered a personal and professional trip down memory lane. I first met Laura at a conference in 2009 having been introduced by Dr JJ Reilly who was already building a team to address the rise in prevalence of child obesity in Scotland and across the globe. With both of us having originally qualified as paediatric dietitians, we exchanged ideas about approaches to clinical care regarding nutrition and weight management for families, research results and collaborated on systematic reviews and educational texts. At that time, obesity among children and adolescents was certainly recognised, but less was known about effectiveness of approaches to treatment, particularly regarding nutrition and less still about the importance of a wholistic approach to management.

Laura has invited guest authors to share their own professional experiences in writing some chapters jointly. Throughout the text she has incorporated comments from her conversations with these other health professionals working in this field, and their extensive experience provides valuables insight and advice for others working with children and families.

This book aims to support practitioners working in fields that intersect with development of healthy weight and growth among children, including dietitians, nutritionists, exercise physiologists, physiotherapists, psychologists, social workers, physicians, teachers and others. It will interest students of these professions as well as practicing clinicians. It reviews the current evidence and best practice while delving into the practical delivery of clinical management and touch on the whole systems agenda.

Dr Laura Stewart is the perfect person to write this book. With 40 years' experience as a clinical dietitian, she has been a tireless advocate for improving nutrition and weight-related health for children and families for over two decades. Dr Laura Stewart was awarded her PhD from the Division of Developmental Medicine, Medical Faculty, University of Glasgow, in 2008, for her PhD thesis on dietetic management of childhood obesity. Laura is recognised as a UK expert on the dietetic management of childhood obesity. She has published many peer-reviewed articles and chapters in medical textbooks on this subject and is an invited member of the Scottish Public Health Network (ScotPHN)'s subgroup the Scottish Public Health Obesity Special Interest Group (SPHOSIG). Dr Stewart was professional adviser to the Scottish Government on the Prevention, Early Detection, Early Intervention Type 2 Diabetes

Framework for Scotland, Diet and Healthy Weight Team. She was also an advisor on the Scottish Government on recommendations on child healthy weight programmes in Scotland (2014), the review of the Scottish Obesity Route Map (2015) and until 2018 was an active member of the Scottish Healthy Weight Pathway working group, Diabetes Group's Diabetes Prevention subgroup and Healthy Weight Leads Network.

She is the right person to bring the authors together in this book to help their experiences with others in this important area.

This book will be an important resource for parents, carers, health professionals, teachers and those who work with children broadly. In writing these chapters, Dr Stewart aims to empower a new generation of professionals in this field.

The book starts with a brief history of methods used to define obesity in young people and summarises what is known about health and psychological impacts of excess adiposity.

Chapter 2 acknowledges the wicked relationship between socio-economic factors and multigenerational obesity prevalence, an issue which still requires stronger policy action in most countries if the adverse consequences are to be prevented. The discussion of hypotheses and theoretical models that have attempted the global rise in obesity prevalence will be important reading for those new to the field of obesity to gain insight into the factors that have coalesced at this time in history that promote storage of excessive body fat.

Chapter 4 is a must read for all, and especially those working clinically with families. It provides a comprehensive discussion of raising the issue of child weight status with families, an area that health professionals will agree needs to be performed with sensitivity, respect and support in order to create supportive, non-stigmatising healthcare and where appropriate, treatment plans. The list of strategies parents found helpful when the topic was raised will be very important to guide discussions.

This book confirms this importance of ensuring health professionals and those working with children have access to current, high-quality continuing professional development in all areas related to child and adolescent obesity and strategies for promotion of healthy lifestyles and healthy growth.

It is important to be aware of resources available locally for families, careers and available for use by to local organisations, as well and regional clinical pathways for treatment.

There are dedicated chapters for specific aspects of lifestyle such as nutrition and physical activity, as well as chapters dedicated to the specific life stages of childhood and adolescence, including those with special needs or disability. While this information is of utmost importance, the chapters on changing behaviour, family meals and measuring and monitoring in practice provide the guidance to implement the learnings from the book.

Importantly the chapters on safeguarding provide an alert to key issues that need to be addressed when supporting development of healthy weight and weight-related health outcomes for children and adolescents. The chapter on systems thinking provides a sobering reminder that no country has yet managed to reverse the relentless rise in the prevalence of obesity, despite many developing policies, strategic plans and blueprints. There is a clear need for implementation of whole of system approaches. This needs to be accompanied by evaluation of both effectiveness and impact, as well as funding to refine programs based on evaluation results. This will help to conserve healthcare resources and ensure the most successful approaches are adopted at scale, such that every child can access the right care in the right place at the right time. This is needed to allow them and their families and carers to thrive.

Clare Collins

Laureate Professor of Nutrition

and Dietetics, The University of Newcastle,

NSW, Australia

Abbreviations

Below is a list of abbreviations used throughout this text book. The full terms are written out only once in this book and then the abbreviation is used in subsequent chapters.

AAP	American Academy of Pediatrics
ABLe-Change	Above and Below Line Change
ACE	Adverse Childhood Experiences
ADHD	Attention-deficit hyperactivity disorder
AHWP	Amsterdam Healthy Weight Programme
ARFID	Avoidant/restrictive food intake disorder
ASD	Autistic spectrum disorder
AYPH	The Association for Young People's Health
BED	Binge eating disorder
BMI	Body Mass Index
BOGOF	Buy-one-get-one-free
BOMSS	British Obesity and Metabolic Surgery Society
CAMH	Children and Adolescent Mental Health
CDP	Chronic Disease Prevention
CMOs	Chief medical officers
COMPACT	Childhood Obesity Modelling for Prevention and Community Transformation
CT	Computer tomography
CV	Cardiovascular
CVD	Cardiovascular disease
CYP	Children and young people/child and young person
DEXA	Dual-energy X-ray absorptiometry
EAR	Estimated average requirements
ECPO	European Coalition of People Living with Obesity
EDNP	Energy-dense nutrient poor
EE	Emotional eating
ENCOMPASS	Evaluation of Programmes in Complex Adaptive Systems
EPODE	Ensemble Prévenons l'Obésité Des Enfants' (*Together Let's Prevent Childhood Obesity*)
GOOS	Genetics of Obesity Study
GRADE	Grading of Recommendations Assessment, Development and Evaluation
HbA1c	Glycated haemoglobin
HCP	Health Care Professional
HFSS	High in fat, sugar and salt

H&SCP	Health and Social Care Professional
HOMA	Homeostatic Model Assessment
ICAD	International Children Accelerometery Database
IGF-1	Insulin-like growth factor-1
IH	Insurance hypothesis
IMD	Indices of Multiple Deprivation
IOTF	International Obesity Task Force
NAFLD	Non-alcoholic fatty liver disease
NASH	Non-alcoholic steatohepatitis
NCD	Non-communicable diseases
NCD-RisC	NCD Risk Factor Collaboration
NCMP	National Child Measurement Programme
NDNS	National diet and nutritional survey
NHANES	National Health and Nutrition Examination Survey
NICE	National Institute for Clinical Excellence
NIHR	National Institute for Health and Care Research
NSS	Non-sugar sweeteners
MASH	Multi agency safeguarding hubs
MC4R	Melanocortin 4 receptor
MDT	Multi-disciplinary team
MEND	Mind, Exercise, Nutrition, Do It
METs	Metabolic equivalents
MPVA	Moderate to vigorous activity
MRI	Magnetic resonance imaging
OECD	Organisation for Economic Cooperation and Development
OSFED	Other specified feeding or eating disorder
PA	Physical activity
PAQ-A	Physical Activity Questionnaire for Adolescents
PAQ-C	Physical Activity Questionnaire for Older Children
PCOS	Polycystic ovarian syndrome
PEC	Picture Exchange Communication
POMC	Propeptide proopiomelanocortin
PHE	Public Health England
PHS	Public Health Scotland
PREM	Patient reported experience measures
PROMS	Patient reported outcome measures
RCPCH	Royal College of Paediatricians and Child Health
RCT	Randomised controlled trials
REM	Ripple Effects Mapping
SAMHSA	Substance Abuse and Mental Health Services Administration
SEIFA	Socio-Economic Indexes for Areas
SEND	Special educational needs and disabilities
SES	Socio-economic status

SHANARRI	Safe, Healthy, Achieving, Nurtured, Active, Respected, Responsible, Included
SIGN	Scottish Intercollegiate Guideline Network
SIMD	Scottish Indices of Multiple Deprivation
SLA	Service level agreement
SMART	Specific, Measurable, Achievable, Recorded, Time-phased
SSB	Sugar sweetened beverages
SUS	Shape Up Somerville
TEI	Total energy intake
TV	Television
UK	United Kingdom
UNICEF	United Nations International Children's Emergency Fund
US	United States
WHO	World Health Organization
WHOSTOPS	Whole of Systems Trial of Prevention Strategies for Childhood Obesity
WSA	Whole systems approach

Acknowledgements

I would like to give a huge thank you to both Dr Clare Neilson and Dr Thomas Stewart for their exceedingly helpful advice reviewing the content and structure of this book. They helped to give me feedback on each chapter and on the overall book contents. Thank you both for your hard work. Without a doubt, many thanks to the authors of the 'guest' chapters and Clare Collins for her gracious foreword.

Therese Stewart and Thomas Stewart both transcribed the recorded interviews with professional practitioners, undertaken for this book. The introduction chapter could not have been written without this important step, so thank you both. This leads me to thank all the practitioners who agreed to have a recorded conversation with me. Your contribution via these conversations has been of great benefit to the overall sense of this book.

Chin Wai Yip spent a ten-week internship with me in 2021 as part of her Nutrition course at Abertay University. During this time, she kick started the literature review for this book. I thank her and wish her all the best for her future career in nutrition.

My last thanks are to the team at Wiley for being so supportive, many thanks.

Laura Stewart
August 2024

Introduction
The Voices of Lived Experience

Laura Stewart

Introduction

The aim of this book is to support healthy weight practitioners such as dietitians, nutritionists, psychologists, social workers, physicians, health coaches and other professionals who currently, or indeed wish to, work in the field of childhood obesity and weight management. It will interest students of these professions as well as practicing clinicians. It explores current evidence and best practice while delving into the practical delivery of clinical management and touches on prevention by briefly looking at the whole systems agenda and the early years.

In this introductory chapter, the points of view of children and young people, their parents and carers are given through a synthesis of published qualitative research of interviews with children and young people living with obesity and their parents. It is intended that giving such insight into the lived experience of children and young people and their families, at the beginning of a text book on childhood obesity and weight management, will be thought provoking for the reader. This introductory chapter is intended to aid weight management practitioners in considering their own personal approaches when reading the subsequent chapters, which cover the science, evidence and best practice of this discipline. This has been put into an introductory chapter to emphasise the importance to practitioners of hearing the voice of lived experienced. All direct quotes from children, young people and parents in this section are taken from and referenced to the original published work.

It was an important concept at the outset of writing this book that the voice of the children and young people living with obesity and their parents was heard and was at the forefront of the reader's mind. Although not the only source, a number of the works quoted below are from published qualitative works by this author and colleagues.

Child and Adolescent Obesity: A Practical Approach to Clinical Weight Management,
First Edition. Edited by Laura Stewart.
© 2024 John Wiley & Sons Ltd. Published 2024 by John Wiley & Sons Ltd.

Another important resource for this section was the recent work undertaken in 2022 by The Association for Young People's Health (AYPH) for NHS England [1].

To give another perspective, this book also brings to the fore the views of experienced professionals working in the field of childhood weight management. A number of one-to-one semi-structured conversations were carried out with clinical and research experts in this field by this author between 2021 and 2023. These included experienced dietitians, service managers, public health practitioners, physical activity experts and psychologists. Rich, unique insights with quotes and discussions of important themes that emerged during these conversations are given below in the second section.

The Voice of Children, Young People Living with Obesity and Their Parents

When Do Parents Look for Support?

For many parents, recognising the need to seek help for their child's weight management is a difficult process. Work by Gillespie et al. found that for some parents even discussing the topic of weight was overwhelming: *'the problem is too big', 'I can't bear to raise it, and I don't want to make things worse'* [2].

Discussing what their reasons for seeking support for their child's weight were, this group of parents described possible 'triggers' for seeking help including

- recognising that their child was being bullied
- being aware that their child was wearing outsized clothes for their age
- having concerns about their child's current or future health [2].

Not being able to recognise that their child's weight was outside the healthy weight zone was something that parents spoke about.

'I didn't realise he was so overweight, I didn't realise he was that, because he doesn't look it because he's broad, so he carries it well, but I was quite shocked to find out his actual weight' [3]. This can lead to difficult conversations happening with health professionals who are raising the topic for the first time. While Murtagh et al. reported that young people can be aware of the need for support with their weight and are actually waiting for their parents to take action, *'I knew about it but my parents didn't believe me'* [4].

Studies reported that consideration of the matter of a child's weight can be overwhelming for parents, *'the problem is too big'* and *'I can't bear to raise it, and I don't want to make things worse'* [2]. Rigby noted that the young people could also feel overwhelming, *'time to comprehend so you don't get overwhelmed'* [1].

Attitudes and Qualities of the Health Professional

Families report that the attitudes of health professionals, especially their ability to build and develop rapport, are important to them [5]. Parents in studies have talked about the necessary qualities of the professional as *'being friendly, supportive, helpful, good listeners, non-judgemental and non-patronising'* [1, 2]. As well as how vital it is that they are seen within a non-stigmatising service [2].

The 2022 work from AYPH discussed the negative feeling that can emerge when professionals do not have the right communication and people skills, *'One hospital appointment made my child feel set for self-destruction'* [1]. Stewart et al. found that professionals not trained in the use of behavioural change techniques found it harder to form a rapport and make the families feel supported [5].

> *'I don't really think it was a success 'cause I don't think we both actually liked the dietitian, em. I think that wasn't just me, he didn't like her'* and *'I expected more than just talk'* [5].

Using Behavioural Change Tools

When it came to aspects of behavioural change tools being used in programmes, it was reported by parents that tools were positive and enabling an improvement in self-esteem and ownership for the child and young person. *'None of us like to be told to do things and so it was like forming a partnership and it worked'* and *'if she wanted a treat of chocolate throughout the day, she had to decide, she has to tell me'* [5].

Using the tool of self-monitoring through keeping a lifestyle diary was seen as helpful in raising awareness of current behaviours, *'I was happy for C to watch TV but I wasn't aware of how much time she was actually watching but when we recorded it I was really surprised. I just wasn't aware of things that is why recording was so good'* [5].

Stigma and Self-esteem

Many studies talked about participants reporting stigmatisation, low self-esteem and bullying of young people living with obesity [1, 6].

> *'he gets bullied, and everything, low self-esteem, he's got no friends, he doesn't go out'* [2].

> *'if my daughter felt better about herself, she wouldn't be so
> angry all the time, she's got quite a lot of emotional issues due
> to being a bit heavy'* [2].

> *'People call me names because they think it's funny but
> it's not'* [4].

For young people, they felt that health services should give equal consideration to their mental health and well-being as to their physical health [1, 7]. Indeed, an important theme emerging from Yerges et al. was titled *'health is like a physical, mental and social balance'*. Their work suggested that weight management programmes need to have a holistic-person-centred approach, taking equally into account these three interlinked aspects of a young person and their family's live [7].

> *'Because I mean like anything that affects a person's like
> day-to-day life I think could fall under health care, whether
> it is physical or mentally'* [7].

A number of studies reported that parents were aware, and anxious, about the emotional effect of their child's weight. They talked about wishing for their child to be happy and how important it is to them, as parents, for their child's self-esteem to be positively impacted by the programme [1, 2].

> *'she used to be embarrassed at school cause there were things
> she couldn't do in PE that she can do now'* [5].

> *'He used to wear jogging bottoms for comfort, but we managed
> to get him dress (in) trousers for school. He was saying it's
> really good isn't it, it has been really good for him'* [3].

Programme Outcomes

This leads to consider what it is that children, young people and their parents regard as a desired outcome of treatment. For those children, young people and the parents interviewed, they reported that concentrating on a weight outcome of treatment was not always a positive concept. There was a reported ambivalence from young people towards being weighed and comments that interactions should be more than just about the number on the scales [7].

> *'Some days, weight is just a number, and then some day's
> weight is something that is weighing me down'* [7].

Informal Support

Yerges et al. noted that although the young people felt able to discuss their knowledge of a 'healthy lifestyle': they knew that they should 'eat healthier' and 'take more' physical exercise, and they struggled to *'actualise these health ideals'* [7]. This is an interesting point which suggests that there is a need for support for problem-solving and developing realistic goals for making day-to-day lifestyle behaviour changes.

The benefit of informal support from others in the kinship circle was reported and from their peers in the weight management peer group [1].

> *'To do it alone and without support can mean we go back into our old ways'* [1], *while 'Being able to see what others can do and that I can do it too if I try hard enough'* [1], *and 'I don't think I would have carried on if ... my friend ... wasn't there'* [1].

What was seen as supportive and important was a person-centred approach that was tailored to the child and young person's needs, *'need to encourage them to take on at their own pace, more likely to achieve'* [1].

The importance of family-based programmes which encourage parental and kinship support is underlined by quotes from young people not feeling supported by the families.

> *'since I do not buy the groceries I have no control over what we have in the house'* [8].

> *'some people in my family, they motivate me to eat well. Then, a couple of days later, they'll start eating the wrong things and they'll try to feed me it and try to make me eat it, and I'm trying to stay healthy in all things. They just keep switching back and forth'* [8].

Potential Barriers

A major barrier cited to achieving lifestyle change goals was eating behaviours, especially around non-hunger eating and having access to easily available high-energy foods [8]. This could be worsened when trying to fit in with peer groups [7, 8].

> *'You're not gonna be like, oh, let me eat a salad while all my friends are eating pizza or whatever, you know?'* [8].

The other potential barriers to change cited by the young people and their parents was bullying and the fear of bullying [1]. In addition to the pressures of life such as school work, exams, keeping up with their peers and social pressure, *'[I feel] different and terrible, like I'm not like everyone else'* [1, 4].

In a study where only females were interviewed, they talked of embarrassment around physical activities and not knowing what or how to do activities [8]. Other studies mention that young people spoke of wanting a 'safe environment' to undertake physical activity [1, 9].

> *'Doing sports around people who are physically healthier than you can cause a lot of anxiety and it takes a lot of help to get rid of that anxiety'* [1].

The Voice of Practitioners Working with Children and Young People Living with Obesity

Most of the conversations with practitioners took place virtually, with a few conducted in person. They all took around one-and-a-half hours. The conversations were recorded and then transcribed in full. A framework analysis approach was used to allow themes and concepts to emerge from the transcribed conversations [10]. The outputs from these conversations are unique to this book and have not been published elsewhere.

A qualitative-type semi-structured script was used as the starting point of the conversations. Some questions were asked as standard for all the participants, while some were pertinent to their particular field and/or profession. While the script was a starting point for discussion, the conversations developed organically following the responses and thoughts of each practitioner. These took place with an understanding of the participants remaining anonymous and none of the quotes in this section are referenced.

Key Advice for New Practitioners

All participants were asked *'what would be the key piece of advice you would wish to give to a new practitioner in the field of childhood weight management'*. From this question, three significant themes stood out; these are outlined in Table I.1. Participants acknowledged that while this was a challenging area to work in, it was also rewarding.

Analysis of all the conversations added a further six themes. These nine themes are now briefly summarised and illustrated with quotes.

Person Centred

The importance of taking a person-centred, holistic approach and not a 'the professional knows best' approach was emphasised by the participants.

Table I.1 Emergent key themes for new participants and quotes.

Themes	Participant quotes
Complexity	*'It is so so complex. And they need to have an understanding of the challenges that are for all families, but particularly for those that are maybe in more deprived areas, who are more vulnerable to the obesogenic environment'.*
Relationships	*'The importance of developing good relationships with the people you are working with and also with your team members, and having that mutual respect and understanding for each other, Being able to learn from each other and deliver messages by learning from each other is really key'.*
Person centred	*'You need to look at the whole perceptive in order to effectively fully understand what is right for that child'.*

'You need to spend the time fully understanding the child and the circumstances of the family. And when I say fully understanding, it is not just diet, it is not just activity. It is understanding the social context, the psycho-social context, the mental health'.

'To take that person centred approach, to not be judgemental, not be didactic, but to explore first. To get permission, understand the family environment and that wider setting. It is not just about education; it is about that wider psychological change. It is not just about what we do or what we eat. But how we do these things and how it fits together'.

'Getting to know the child. Exploring the child's world. The social dynamics, their routine, food choices. Don't just jump into advice, get to know them. Work out what you can tailor to that individual. It's not simple and you might get your information over multiple appointments'.

Challenges and Complexity

The complexities of childhood obesity and its management was returned to time and again as a major challenge for any practitioner. The complexities discussed varied from family dynamics and circumstances, the obesogenic environment, the underlying psycho-social components and societal attitudes to children and young people living with obesity.

'By complexity, I mean the family dynamic, the social circumstances and sometimes underlying disabilities or additional needs that child might have'.

> *'It's so multi-factorial, it's so not down to individual choice, it's so wrapped up into politics and social norms and beliefs and values'.*

> *'In reality it is such a complex, multi-component condition. And it is a condition that people are living with, experiencing with not just physical but psychological and social, daily impacts. So, we really need a bio-social model to be able to deliver the care people need'.*

Relationships

Relationships came up in every conversation. From the point of view of the practitioner, these relationships were between themselves and the child and young person and their parents, the team and possible gate-keepers (a term for those who refer into the service). This concept of relationships is mapped out in Table I.2.

Rapport

The need for the practitioner to be approachable and have the ability to establish and develop rapport was a strong sub-theme of relationships.

> *'It's about the importance of establishing rapport, the importance of having a relationship with the family whereby you can start. Having empathy with them and showing that you can understand the position, or circumstance they are in, to enable you to work with them and for them to have the trust in you is quite important as well. And that can sometimes take a lot of time'.*

> *'But I genuinely think that being open and honest with the families is important to building that rapport'.*

Parenting

A further sub-theme of relationships was characterised in the thematic analysis as 'parenting'. This included both the role of parents in supporting their child and also the act of parenting.

> *'I think with that, with food as well, it is all about role modelling. It's so important. If you have got a parent that goes out on that Sunday run, they do it without fail. That is important role modelling for a child'.*

> *'For those patterns to change or to be challenged can be very difficult. I think it is important we don't place sole responsibility on the young person. It is expected their parents will be part of that process'.*

Table I.2 Mapping of relationships with the practitioner.

	– Child/young person (CYP)	*'It can take them a while to open up to a healthcare professional, having the consistency and seeing the same person, being able to build on that relationship, helps them open up and it's a bit more of two-way street when you are negotiating things'.*
	– Parents	*'Helping to manage the parents' frustrations, which, you know, are concerns. And not look, and that's where it comes back, I suppose to the behavioural to the parenting side of it, and not looking reinforce these behaviours but helping the family, the parents to manage them and have boundaries'.*
Practitioner's relationships to	– CYP and parents	*'For those patterns to change or to be challenged can be very difficult. I think it is important we don't place sole responsibility on the young person. It is expected their family will be part of that process'.*
	– The team	*'I say inter-professional rather than multi-disciplinary deliberately. Because sometimes I feel you can have a multi-disciplinary team that functions separately to one another. When you are dealing with obesity you really want to be dealing with all of those different aspects together'.*
	– Gatekeepers	*'Likewise for the school nurses, likewise for the health visitors. Because I think sometimes that training either exists as a one off at the start and then never gets refreshed and clued up. And I think these people need to be on regular refresher training on growth, nutrition, feeding advice, as a general thing'.*

The Team

The participants included those who had worked within a formal multidisciplinary team (MDT) and a uni profession (usually) dietetic-led weight management service. This led to rich and varied points of view on the role teams play in supporting both individual practitioners and the children and young people they work with.

> *'The person who that family have really clicked with. You decide in those first assessments, who is the priority area for that family. Is it that you really need to be focussing on the social side of things? So, the social worker is the person who you really need to be moving through the stages of change? Then bringing in some expert advice from the rest of the team'.*

> *'It is important the team can understand that, that we are all working towards the same goal. That being informed by the family, but also supporting the team with aspects of training. We support each other'.*

Psychologist

The role of a psychologist was understood by participants to be fundamental in supporting weight management, behaviour change and mental well-being for children and young people. Best practice was considered to be a psychologist embedded within a team, with at the very least a good working relationship with the local psychology service. Access to informal discussions with psychologist was considered to be valuable in supporting up skilling practitioners and with reflective practice.

> *'I think it is crucial for the psychologist to be embedded within the team so they can learn from everybody else in the team and everybody else can learn from them'.*

> *'Psychology is key. That might be our tier three families who are that bit more complex and have more additional needs. They might need that psychology. If not a specific child healthy weight psychology, then at least links and pathways into CAMHS (child and adolescent mental health service) to be able to provide that'.*

Stigma

Stigma interfaced and overlapped with a number of other themes, as illustrated in Figure I.1. Stigma here encompasses weight stigma and bias.

> *'If we haven't had the forethought to plan ahead for example, or services haven't got the right equipment that contributes to a young person feeling different and embarrassed. Which is going to affect how they feel about coming back and the conversations that they have'.*

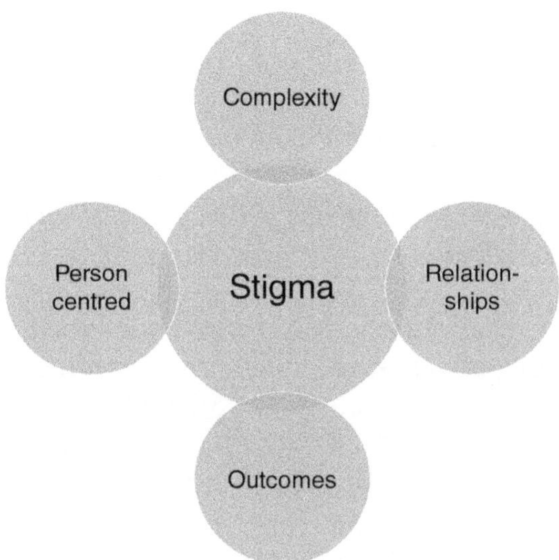

Figure I.1 Interplay of themes with stigma.

'So that then leads me to think about, in terms of society's view, that that is actually one of the most fundamental challenges as well. Because of the stigma that overweight and people living with obesity have. And I think that needs to be addressed as well, and I think it is being addressed'.

'Because a lot of their parents would have had similar experiences. They would have been overweight and obese themselves, and therefore probably have experienced stigma and negative associations with that. And that stays with them, and therefore that makes it difficult for them to seek out support. If they've had a difficult experience, or a negative experience, themselves in addressing their own weight, or perhaps not addressing it and just internalising it, then that then impacts on their child as well. So, I think it is through all layers'.

Outcomes

There was much discourse during the conversations on the need of outcomes (as collected from a service point of view) to be person centred and include a mixture of quantifiable and qualitative type data, such as patient stories and patient outcome measures, for example being able to fit into smaller clothes sizes or being able to run for longer or faster.

'The focus from their point of view is the focus on weight can be counter-intuitive and can create stress and pressure. We want to be in a place we can quickly identify those patterns of behaviour and seek additional specialist help'.

*'Often the parents will say they want the child to be healthier.
In terms of physical health and to lose weight. I will always ask
the young person what they want. They would often say words
to that affect. When I ask what that means for them, it might
be about be about keeping up with their peers, running as fast
as them, not getting out of breath, choosing different clothes,
feeling more confident in social situations. Everyone is different'.*

The use of Body Mass Index (BMI) was categorised as a sub-theme
of outcomes. While participants consider collection of weight, height
and thus BMI necessary, they clearly expressed a point of view that it
should not be the only measurement of success for the children and
young people, the parents or the service.

*'For example, I think in younger children when you are
working with them it is things like families eating meals
together. It's these sort of things where sometimes that sort of
thing becomes lost. So, it can be families eating meals together.
I think reducing screen time. If there's more stories going on
in the house. Things like that can be a stepping stone towards
making changes. I actually think I'm, yeah, I'm becoming less
interested in the BMI in outcomes for families'.*

*'If we think about all the different dimensions there, there is
something there about health and well-being part of that and
weight and BMI being one part of that as well. So, I do think
there needs to be more than that. I don't think it can just be
down to BMI'.*

Systems

Systems brought together wider aspects of the world we live in, such as
discussions around the obesogenic environment, interplay of environment
and genetics, targeting early years interventions.

*'So, there's something there about the connection between
working with individual families, but understanding the context
that these families are living in, and getting that balance right
between addressing all of those things that are needing to be'.*

*'And that, to my mind, means starting earlier. If we are
going to have a hope of more effective treatments, or more
successful prevention of adulthood obesity, we need to start our
treatments earlier. I think that's the other thing that has come
out from the evidence, children are coming into treatment*

when it is probably already getting a bit late. Children are coming into treatment when they are already on a particular trajectory of lifestyle behaviours, a particular trajectory of weight and treatment has to start earlier in my view. I think the evidence is pretty clear on that'.

'But I think we are at the point now where we do need to acknowledge that there is something there about genetics as well'.

Programmes

There was strong feeling that childhood weight management programmes should be underpinned by the best available evidence and be structured while at the same time supporting an individualised approach.

'I do think it is helpful to have structured programmes, that you can use. That's consistency from the practitioner's point of view, but also for families who may drop out or re-engage with your service over time, because that happens quite a lot. That they're hearing the same thing'.

'We have to do multiple things at multiple different stages and we will have an impact, accumulatively with all those things'.

'But it's multicomponent. It's more than just educating. You have to be able to achieve the behaviour change or the appropriate behaviour in families. You have to have the psychological component. You have to have interactive teaching, where everything is co-creating what their lifestyle is going to be. It has got to be meaningful for them, something they want to do'.

Eating Behaviours

While all aspects of lifestyle advice/energy balance were discussed eating behaviours stood out as challenging for both the practitioner and the families.

'I suppose around fussy eating and, fussy eating which can then on a continuum become restrictive eating and looking to help to challenge in that area'.

'I think a lot of people assume because they are coming to a weight management clinic, we are going to turn their diet upside down. They are going to have to change everything they

> *eat, but for a lot of young people it might be about portions, or might be about making slight different snack choices. It's actually quantity rather than variety'.*

> *'I find a diet history isn't my preferred method, but I try and do it so its not an interrogation but a chat through the day'.*

Conclusions

It can be seen from both of these sections that there are many similarities between what the young people, their parents and the practitioners consider to be important. All of the points raised in this chapter are explored and expanded on in the chapters of this book.

This book has been written from the point of view of delivering a person-centred, compassionate approach to childhood weight management. It is hoped that this introductory chapter has helped to set the scene from the perspective of those with lived experience. To keep this voice in the readers mind, each chapter commences with a suitable quote.

References

1 Rigby, E., McKoewn, R., and Wortley, L. (2022). The experiences of young people and their families living with excess weight: themes from engagement work. https://ayph.org.uk/wp-content/uploads/2022/04/CEW-Themes-from-engagement-work.pdf (accessed 29 March 2024).

2 Gillespie, J., Midmore, C., Hoeflich, J. et al. (2015). Parents as the start of the solution: a social marketing approach to understanding triggers and barriers to entering a childhood weight management service. *J. Hum. Nutr. Diet.* 28: 83–92. https://doi.org/10.1111/jhn.12237.

3 Stewart, L., Chapple, J., Hughes, A.R. et al. (2008). Parents' journey through treatment for their child's obesity: a qualitative study. *Arch. Dis. Child.* 93: 35–39. https://doi.org/10.1136/adc.2007.125146.

4 Murtagh, J., Dixey, R., and Rudolf, M. (2006). A qualitative investigation into the levers and barriers to weight loss in children: opinions of obese children. *Arch. Dis. Child.* 91: 920–923. https://doi.org/10.1136/adc.2005.085712.

5 Stewart, L., Chapple, J., Hughes, A.R. et al. (2008). The use of behavioural change techniques in the treatment of paediatric obesity: qualitative evaluation of parental perspectives on treatment. *J. Hum. Nutr. Diet.* 21: 464–473. https://doi.org/10.1111/j.1365-277X.2008.00888.x.

6 Hagell, A. and Wortley, L. (2022) The experiences of young people and their families affected by excess weight: evidence from existing research. AYPH

7 Yerges, A.L., Snethen, J.A., and Carrel, A.L. (2021). Adolescent girls with overweight and obesity feel physically healthy and highlight the importance of mental health. *SAGE Open. Nurs.* 7: https://doi.org/10.1177/23779608211018523.

8 Cardel, M.I., Szurek, S.M., Dillard, J.R. et al. (2020). Perceived barriers/facilitators to a healthy lifestyle among diverse adolescents with overweight/obesity: a qualitative study. *Obes. Sci. Pract.* 6: 638–648. https://doi.org/10.1002/osp4.448.

9 Rees, R.W., Caird, J., Dickson, K. et al. (2014). 'It's on your conscience all the time': a systematic review of qualitative studies examining views on obesity among young people aged 12–18 years in the UK. *BMJ Open.* 4: https://doi.org/10.1136/bmjopen-2013-004404.

10 Spencer, L., Ritchie, J., and Lewis, J. et al. (2003). Quality in qualitative evaluation: a framework for assessing research evidence. *Gov Chief Soc Res Off Occas Pap Ser No 2.*

1 What Is Childhood Obesity and Why Does It Matter

Laura Stewart

'The problem is too big'. [1]

Introduction

Managing and securing a sustained decrease in the prevalence of childhood obesity is one of the major public health challenges of the 21st century. In 2021, the World Health Organization (WHO) reported that there were 39 million children under the age of 5 living with overweight or obesity in the year 2020, while there were over 340 million children and young people (CYP)[1] aged 5–19 living with overweight or obesity in the year 2016 [2]. The WHO demonstrated the importance they placed on tackling childhood obesity to worldwide health by setting a target in 2011 for worldwide childhood obesity prevalence to be no more than 2010 levels by the year 2025 [3].

In 2017 the NCD Risk Factor Collaboration (NCD-RisC) looked at the worldwide trends of body mass index (BMI) in CYP from 1975 to 2016. They found an increase in the prevalence of obesity for girls in that time from 0.7% (0.4–1.2) to 5.6% (4.8–6.5). For boys the prevalence increased from 0.9% (0.5–1.3) in 1975 to 7.8% (6.7–9.1) in 2016. The trend in rising CYP's BMI now appears to have levelled out. These raised levels remain in high-income countries, while the prevalence is continuing to increase in certain parts of Asia [4]. There is also evidence to suggest that the COVID-19 lockdowns were associated with a higher rate of increase in BMI compared to the pre-pandemic period [5].

---

[1]Throughout this book the abbreviation CYP is used as short hand for the singular – child and young person, and the plural – children and young people.

Child and Adolescent Obesity: A Practical Approach to Clinical Weight Management,
First Edition. Edited by Laura Stewart.
© 2024 John Wiley & Sons Ltd. Published 2024 by John Wiley & Sons Ltd.

The writing of this book started during the COVID-19 pandemic of 2020–2021, during which there emerged an association between obesity and type 2 diabetes and a higher likelihood of acquiring COVID-19 as well as worse outcomes from the illness including death. While the death risk from COVID-19 was greatest in the older population, it was also seen in younger adults who had higher BMI [6]. This experience further emphasised the need to consider excess weight and high BMIs as health risks. This matters for our consideration of childhood obesity, as will be discussed in this chapter there is a higher likelihood of a young person with obesity becoming an adult living with obesity.

This first chapter seeks to 'set the scene' around how we define obesity in childhood and why this is an important topic in terms of health and socio-psycho consequences. Viewing obesity as a chronic disease, requiring long-term support and management [5] throughout the life course, is the starting position of writing this text book.

Defining Obesity in Childhood

It is important to understand when considering a definition of clinical obesity that it is an excess accumulation of body fat (adipose) that has led to, or has increased the risk of, chronic disease and co-morbidities [7]. There is strong evidence that central visceral fat distribution in children and adolescents is associated with increased health risks [8, 9]. Meaning that the health risk is due to where the excess body fat actually sits within the body and not just the actual amount.

Visceral fat = body fat that is stored within the abdominal cavity and is therefore stored around a number of important internal organs such as the liver, pancreas and intestines.

Co-morbidities associated with excess body fat will include:

- Cardiovascular disease
- Insulin resistance
- Pre-diabetes
- Type 2 diabetes
- Dyslipidaemia
- Hypertension
- Psychological and social morbidity
- Asthma
- Impaired fertility
- Orthopaedic problems, e.g. in the hips and ankles

- Breathing problems and sleep apnoea
- Fatty liver disease
- Some cancers, e.g. breast, bowel, pancreatic, oesophageal and gallbladder
- Acceleration of puberty in both girls and boys
- Persistence of obesity into adulthood [10, 11]

Regardless of age, we cannot tell if someone has overweight or obesity simply by looking at them. Being able to accurately measure total body fat and its distribution is not practical from a routine perspective. Total body fat can be measured using dual-energy X-ray absorptiometry (DEXA) scan [5]; however, the DEXA scan cannot measure visceral fat accurately. While, accurate measurements of visceral fat can be made using computer tomography (CT) and magnetic resonance imaging (MRI) [12].

Therefore, the 'easy to use' proxy measurement of BMI is widely used for day-to-day clinical practice in childhood weight management. While the calculation of BMI in childhood is the same as for adults, the dynamic growth and changes in body fat seen during growth require it to be plotted on an age- and sex-related BMI centile chart [5, 13].

Body Mass Index

$$BMI = weight\,(kg) \div height\,(m)^2$$

The use of BMI to categorise childhood overweight and obesity requires clinical relevance of this proxy measurement of body fat. That is at what level of BMI is there a significant increase in the adverse health consequences of childhood overweight and obesity [14–16]. A cut off with a high specificity has generally been regarded as more important for clinical applications than a high sensitivity to avoid unnecessarily classifying some children as having obesity [5, 17, 18].

Specificity = The proportion of negatives correctly identified by the test.

Sensitivity = The proportion of positives correctly identified by the test [19].

BMI in children rises steadily in the period following birth and then drops during the pre-school years. It then subsequently slowly increases during childhood until adulthood. Adiposity rebound is the term used to describe the point when the BMI starts to rise again after the lowest point.

Evidence suggests that the earlier the age of adiposity rebound is associated with an increased risk of later obesity in childhood [20, 21]. Due to this changing curve of BMI during childhood and in differences between male and female, BMI needs to be plotted on a national specific, sex appropriate BMI centile chart and from this a weight category can be made.

BMI Centile Charts

For some years the diagnosis of obesity has been based on the cut-off point of the 95th centile, with the 85th centile taken as the cut off for overweight, first on the United States' (US) National Health and Nutrition Examination Surveys (NHANES) charts and then on other national BMI centile charts. It was considered that children with a BMI over the 95th centile had a higher risk of persistence of obesity in adulthood and of obesity-related diseases [16, 22]. This cut-off point had been noted by Himes and Dietz as having a high specificity and a moderate to high sensitivity [16].

Discussion of BMI and BMI charts is returned to in depth in Chapter 8. At this point it is worth noting that in the United Kingdom (UK), the WHO/UK 1990 BMI centile charts should be used. Unlike other countries in the UK, there are essentially two definitions with different BMI centile cut-off points used:

For **clinical** work, the ≥98th BMI centile for defining obesity is used, with the ≥91st BMI centile used for overweight. For **epidemiology** work, the ≥95th BMI centile for defining obesity is used, with the ≥85th BMI centile used for overweight [13, 23].

Fat Distribution and Waist

We have discussed above the importance of excess body fat and central distribution to the increased risk of disease, co-morbidities and ill health. Measurement of waist as an indicator of increased visceral fat and thus an increased risk of particularly cardiovascular disease (CVD) and type 2 diabetes has been used in adults for some time [7]. While in CYP there has been evidence supporting that the waist circumference measurement is a useful tool for measuring fat distribution, and particularly for identifying central fatness [8, 24], there has been a fluctuating use of waist measurements in clinical practice.

One of the main reasons for this is the perceived difficult in taking the measurement, including embarrassment for the CYP, and a norm comparison to use. For example, previously in the UK waist circumference centiles were available on the back of BMI centile charts [25].

Recent evidence in CYP waist-to-height ratio has been shown to correlate well with the risk of co-morbidities, in particular the increased risk of CVD [26–28]. The figure of 0.5 or above is considered to be an indication of increased risk for all age groups and genders. We will return to waist and taking measurements in Chapter 8.

$$\text{Waist} - \text{Height ratio} = \text{waist measurement (in cms) divided by the height measurement (in cms)}.$$

Aetiology of Obesity

Before going further with a consideration of why childhood obesity is a topic that matters, we should turn to the aetiology of weight gain and obesity. Weight gain and the increasing prevalence of obesity across the global is multi-faceted. An excellent report that examined and high-lighted the complexities around obesity is the UK's Foresight report from 2007 [29]. Figure 1.1 is a simplified graphic of the complex mapping of interacting positive and negative influences on individuals and society on energy balance explored by Foresight (07-1179-obesity-building-system-map.pdf (`publishing.service.gov.uk`)). The Foresight Report is returned to in Chapter 3.

When seeing individual CYP and their families, there is a need to consider a whole person approach and those influences over which they

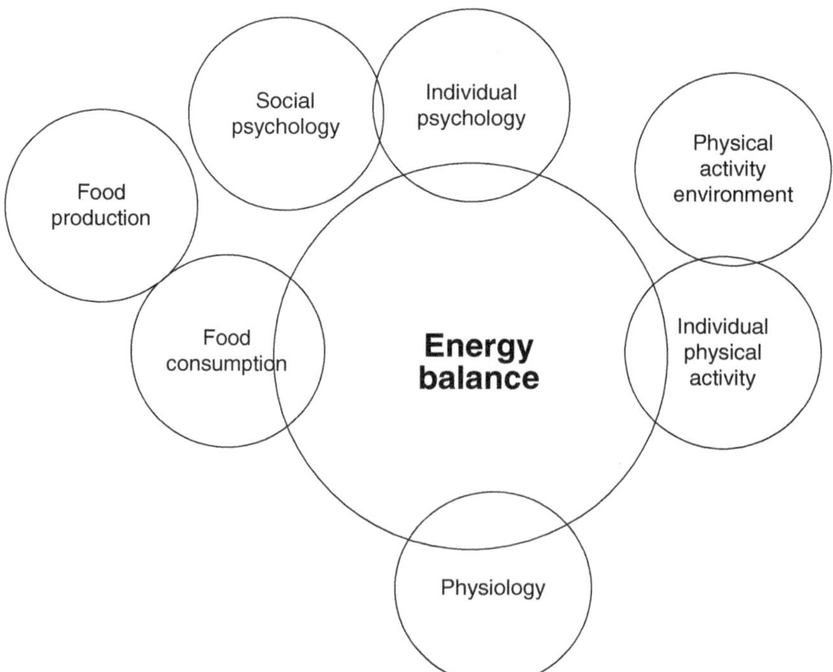

Figure 1.1 Simplified foresight mapping.
Source: Adapted from Butland et al. [29].

may have no control. Foresight indicates us that we must take the holistic approach by viewing and considering:

- *'Biology*
- *Impact of early life and growth patterns*
- *Behaviour*
  - *Food intake and activity behaviours*
  - *What motivates people's decisions and choices?*
- *The living environment*
  - *Technology*
  - *Opportunities for physical activity*
  - *Food and drink access availability*
- *Economic drivers of food production and consumption*
  - *The price of food and drink*
  - *Food marketing*
  - *Purchasing capacity and impact on eating patterns*
  - *Impact of work practices' [29].*

While reading about the individual aspects of energy balance and using behavioural change tools in clinical management as well as considering the chapter on whole systems approach, keep this complexity in the forefront of your mind.

Polygenetics

Much research has been undertaken into the identification of possible genes that could influence human obesity phenotypes. While considerable work has been carried out, mainly through the study of mice, research into genetics and human obesity suggests that there are a number of genes or their variants, which could influence the development of human obesity – polygenetics [30–32]. For polygenetic obesity, it has been suggested that the most common genetic causes are a number of genes which could 'predispose' a person to gaining excess fat leading to obesity if they were exposed to an environment which encourages the necessary behaviours, i.e. high fat diet, low levels of activity [30, 31]. Indeed studies have identified 32 loci that are of significance in pre-disposing an individual to obesity [5].

It has been suggested that by identifying common gene variants that predispose individuals to obesity subgroups of people with obesity could be targeted for particular interventions such as specific diets, behavioural approaches or drugs [32]. In polygenetic obesity research, many genes and variations of genes have been investigated for possible influence on the development of obesity these include those in food regulation, energy expenditure, and lipid and carbohydrate metabolism.

Monogenetics

Although rare, monogenetic causes of obesity in CYP will sometimes be seen in a childhood weight management service. The Genetics of Obesity Study (GOOS) based at the University of Cambridge, in the UK (Home – Genetics of Obesity Study (goos.org.uk)), has conducted significant work in this area [31–33]. The GOOS study has led to the identification of seven monogenetic causes of obesity [32]. Most of these have involved mutations in propeptide proopiomelanocortin (POMC), melanocortin 4 receptor (MC4R) and the hormone leptin. These are all involved in appetite regulation and energy balance within the hypothalamus [31, 32].

Mutations in MC4R are believed to be found in approximately 3–5% of people with a BMI above 40. Mutations in MC4R display a range of phenotypes including showing no signs of obesity to severe obesity particularly at an early age. They also include individuals showing hyperphagia and hyperinsulinaemia while having increased lean body mass and linear growth [31, 33, 34].

Deficiencies in the hormone leptin have been reported to produce extreme obesity, again usually from a young age. With increased appetite, hyperphagia and hypogonadotropic hypogonadism, injections of leptin in these individuals can reverse the hyperphagia and extreme obesity [31].

POMC is a propeptide involved in appetite control, energy balance, and in skin pigmentation, adrenal function. Individuals with POMC mutations are reported as having severe obesity from an early age, hyperphagia, altered pigmentation, usually red hair, and adrenal insufficiency [31, 34].

Inheritable Disorders

There are several inheritable disorders in which obesity is a clinical feature of the syndrome and therefore need to be mentioned here. Lobstein et al. suggested around 30 such inherited disorders; most of these are associated with a level of a learning disabilities and dysmorphic features. The most common inherited disorders seen in routine childhood weight management clinical practice will be:

- Down's syndrome
- Prader-Willi syndrome
- Duchenne muscular dystrophy
- Fragile X [35].

Many of these individuals will be seen in specialist clinics and working with CYP with special needs is explored further in Chapter 13.

Endocrine Causes of Obesity

The endocrine glands produce hormones that are important in the regulation and maintenance of a stable body environment. In children they are particularly important in ensuring normal growth and the timing of puberty. There are a number of endocrine disorders caused by dysfunction in the production of hormones or their utilisation that are associated with childhood obesity. These include hypothyroidism, growth hormone insufficiency, hypopituitarism, hypogonadotrophic hypogonadism, excessive corticosteroid administration, pseudohypoparathyroidism and craniopharyngioma [36].

Many of these endocrine disorders and the inheritable syndromes discussed above manifest short stature as a clinical feature [36, 37]. There is strong agreement that in clinical practice obesity in children who present with short stature for their age should be referred to a tertiary paediatric centre for further investigation for possible underlying medical causes of their obesity.

Adverse Childhood Experiences and Childhood Obesity

Adverse childhood experiences (ACEs) are described as *'potentially traumatic events that occur in childhood and adolescence'* [38]. ACEs could include any of the following:

- Physical abuse
- Sexual abuse
- Emotional abuse
- Living with someone who abused drugs
- Living with someone who abused alcohol
- Exposure to domestic violence
- Living with someone who has gone to prison
- Living with someone with serious mental illness
- Losing a parent through divorce, death or abandonment
- Traumatic weight related experiences (such as bullying related to weight) [38]

Experiences of one of multiple ACEs have been found to be associated with a number of conditions in later life such as CVD and cancers. While there is evidence to show that ACEs are also associated with a higher risk of overweight or obesity for CYP [5, 39, 40]. ACEs are returned to and discussed in more depth in Chapter 12.

Why Childhood Obesity Matters

CYP obesity matters because of the increased risk of health as well as the psychosocial consequences. An excellent, and still relevant, paper written on childhood obesity is by Lobstein et al., and this lists the medical consequences (psychosocial consequences are discussed later in this chapter) of obesity in CYP as:

- Pulmonary
  - Sleep apnoea
  - Asthma
  - Pickwickian syndrome
- Orthopaedic
  - Slipped capital epiphyses
  - Blount's disease (tibia vara)
  - Tibial torsion
  - Cartilage damage in the knee (osteochondritis dissecans)
  - Flat feet
  - Ankle sprains
  - Increased risk of fractures
- Neurological
  - Idiopathic intracranial hypertension (e.g. pseudotumour cerebri)
- Gastroenterological
  - Cholelithiasis
  - Liver steatosis/non-alcoholic fatty liver
  - Gastro-oesophageal reflux
- Endocrine
  - Insulin resistance/impaired glucose tolerance
  - Type 2 diabetes
  - Menstrual abnormalities
  - Polycystic ovary syndrome
  - Hypercorticism
- Cardiovascular
  - Hypertension
  - Dyslipidaemia
  - Fatty streaks
  - Left ventricular hypertrophy
- Other
  - Systemic inflammation/raised C-reactive protein [35, 41].

These increased risks of medical consequences of CYP obesity are due to long-term excess weight and body fat. Freedman et al. concluded that the most significant association between living with obesity in childhood and CVD risk factors in later life were from the tracking of obesity from childhood into adulthood [42]. The evidence overwhelming suggests that CYP living with obesity, particularly adolescents, become adults living with obesity [43, 44]. Dietz noted that approximately 50% of adolescents living with obesity become adults living with obesity including having an increased rate of CVD and diabetes [45]. Onset of obesity before the age of 5 years is seen as a risk factor for obesity in adolescence and later life [46]. A wide ranging and worldwide review by The Global BMI Mortality Collaboration found that a BMI over $25\,kg/m^2$ (for those who had never smoked) was associated with an increased all-cause mortality. The relationship was seen as 'steep' in every region across the globe, apart from South Asia were the numbers of deaths reported as small [47].

Cardiovascular Risk Factors

In 1999 Dietz and Nelson found that 65% of 5–10 years old living with obesity had at least one CVD risk factor and that 25% of the same age group had at least two or more [48]. One of the reports from the Bogalusa Heart Study reported that 59% CYP with a $BMI \geq 99^{th}$ centile (US BMI centile charts) were found to have at least two CVD risk factors [43]. While a systematic review by Reilly et al. cited quality studies reporting an association between childhood obesity and CVD risk factors, including:

- high blood pressure (hypertension)
- dyslipidaemia
- abnormalities in the left ventricular mass and/or function
- hyperinsulinaemia and/or insulin resistance [49].

The Metabolic Syndrome

The metabolic syndrome is the name that has been given to a variety of clinical abnormalities that are known to be risk factors for CVD [50, 51].

While there is still some disagreement about the definition of the metabolic syndrome, there is, however, consensus that it should include a combination of the following:

- Insulin resistance/hyperinsulinaemia
- Obesity – particularly central visceral fat distribution
- Dyslipidaemia – high triglycerides, high low-density lipoprotein (LDL) cholesterol, low high-density lipoprotein (HDL) cholesterol
- Impaired glucose tolerance or type 2 diabetes mellitus
- Essential hypertension – increased systolic and diastolic blood pressure
- Polycystic ovary syndrome.

Type 2 Diabetes

Type 2 diabetes was previously seen as a disease of adults, even later adulthood; however, it is now reported in adolescents [35, 52]. With excess body weight and obesity reported as the single most important risk factor for the development of adolescent type 2 diabetes. The American Diabetes Association noted that around 85% of children diagnosed with type 2 diabetes have overweight or obesity [52]. Other risks factors include a family history of type 2 diabetes and ethnicity [35, 53, 54]. There are well reported higher incidences of type 2 diabetes in non-white populations in particular African American, Hispanics, Asians and American Indians [35, 52, 54, 55]. The onset of puberty seems to play a role in the development of type 2 diabetes with diagnosis typically seen over the age of 10 years during middle to late puberty [54].

The early onset of type 2 diabetes in adolescence is of concern as it is believed that it increases the risks of disease complications such as CVD, kidney failure, visual impairment and limb amputation will be seen at an earlier age in adulthood [35, 52]. Although the numbers of children with clinical type 2 diabetes is relatively low, the numbers are without a doubt increasing with the increased levels of obesity prevalence in this age group [35, 52]. A UK report in 2021 looking at CYP aged 0–15 years noted that over 90% of CYP diagnosed with type 2 diabetes were living with obesity at the time of their diagnosis [56].

Insulin Resistance

An important precursor to the development of pre-diabetes and type 2 diabetes is insulin resistance. It is therefore worth taking time at this point to consider what insulin resistance is and why it can be affected by body weight.

Insulin is the hormone required by the body for the cellular uptake of circulating blood glucose [57]. There is a complex relationship between development of hypertension, dyslipidaemia and hyperinsulinaemia. Excess body fat, specifically centrally distributed visceral fat, would appear to cause a decreased sensitivity to the utilisation of insulin in certain cells. Meaning that although the body is producing sufficient insulin, various cells and organs cannot utilise the insulin effectively, which in turn leads to increased circulating glucose. This increased blood glucose in turn stimulates further insulin production, leading to elevated circulating levels of both glucose and insulin.

It is believed that these elevated glucose and insulin levels can cause a disturbance in a number of cycles, which can in some individuals ultimately lead to dyslipidaemia and hypertension. The exact mechanism of how hyperinsulinaemia causes hypertension remains unclear; however, it has been shown in adolescents to be reversible with weight loss and exercise [57]. Viner et al. found that in a weight management clinic of CYP aged 2–18 years that 40% had hyperinsulinism, 11% impaired fasting glucose, while 30% had dyslipidaemia and 32% hypertension [58].

Measuring insulin resistance is possible but exceedingly complicated for routine practice and is typically seen in research studies. The euglycaemic insulin clamp is the gold standard method used in research, where insulin sensitivity (inverse of insulin resistance) is measured by the amount of glucose required to maintain normal glucose levels (i.e. eugylcaemia) during continuous intravenous administration of insulin and glucose [51, 57].

Methods seen in clinical practice include the homeostatic model assessment (HOMA). HOMA is a calculation using fasting plasma insulin multiplied by the fasting plasma glucose then divided by 22.5. Scores range from 0 to 15, the higher the score the greater the insulin resistance [51, 59, 60]. Another method that may be seen in clinical practice utilises fasting C-peptide levels as a proxy measure for insulin, due to C-peptide being produced in the body in equal amounts to insulin [57, 61].

Non-Alcoholic Fatty Liver Disease

Non-alcoholic fatty liver disease (NAFLD) is seen in children and adolescents living with obesity. The term NAFLD is used to describe a range of liver conditions from fatty infiltration of the liver (steatosis), through non-alcoholic steatohepatitis (NASH) to liver cirrhosis [62, 63]. In 2006 Patton et al. suggested that NAFLD that was seen in CYP was significantly different from liver disease that is seen in adults [63]. As with type 2 diabetes, there appears to be a strong association with the development of NAFLD and visceral obesity, insulin resistance and race/ethnicity [62–64]. Many of the CYP with NAFLD may actually be asymptomatic and therefore without a diagnosis unaware of the disease progression. Although diagnosis of NAFLD may vary across the world a diagnosis can be made with persistent high liver function blood tests and with an ultrasound scan of the liver [65]. The progression of the disease has been noted to be slowed down and even reversed by controlling weight and lifestyle changes [35].

Puberty and Polycystic Ovarian Syndrome

Early onset, known as precocious puberty, can be seen in young people living with obesity. Accelerated height growth and hormone imbalances play a role. This can often be destressing for both the young person and their parents.

Polycystic ovarian syndrome (PCOS) is a condition that affects the female menstrual cycle and fertility. It is characterised by a combination of

- High levels of male hormones
- Irregular or no menstrual cycle
- Hirsutism (excessive hair growth)
- Acne
- Small cysts on the ovaries may or may not be present [35, 66].

PCOS is associated with excess weight and insulin resistance in both adolescents and adults. Lobstein et al. note that PCOS is often undiagnosed in adolescents and that the prevalence in this group is unknown.

Respiratory Problems

Sleeping disorders are well recognised in individuals living with obesity, especially with severe obesity [35]. This can include heavy snoring, resistance to airflow and sleep apnoea. Speiser et al. suggest that CYP living with obesity can be up to six times more likely to have an obstructive sleep apnoea compared to similarly aged peers [66]. There has also been a suggestion of an association between the reduction in oxygen flow in the body and the development of insulin resistance.

A number of studies have shown an association between childhood obesity and asthma. However, in their reviews of childhood obesity both Lobstein et al. and Speiser et al. suggest that a causative biological link between asthma and excessive weight should not be assumed to be a bi-directional link [35, 66].

Orthopaedic

CYP living with obesity and overweight have been reported to have a higher risk of developing certain orthopaedic problems such as Blount's disease (a bowing of the legs), flat feet, ankle sprains, slipped epiphysis, osteoarthritis and fractures [35, 66].

Psychosocial

There is no doubt that there is a negative relationship between living with obesity and psychosocial well-being [67]. Weight stigma and bullying are reported in childhood, with complications from these of isolation, disordered eating and self-harm [67]. While in later life lower social, academic and economic attainment is seen for those who lived with overweight and obesity as CYP [35, 68]. For women, but interestingly not for men, adverse psychosocial effects relating to fewer years in education, higher rates of poverty and lower rates of marriage and household income have also been reported. Viner and Cole reporting on a 1970 British birth cohort noted that when childhood obesity persists into adulthood, there is an association with poorer employment and relationship outcomes for women [69].

Weight stigma is defined as negative attitudes and beliefs that devalue people based on their weight status [70].

Weight stigma includes bias, discrimination, stereotyping and social exclusion of a person living with overweight or obesity. Weight stigma by others can in turn become internalised weight stigma which negatively impacts on psychosocial well-being, mood and self-esteem [71]. Experiencing weight stigma can lead to someone of any age group to increase their energy intake and can cause further weight gain. There has also been noted that weight stigma can often lead to the avoidance of health care and physical activity [5], with reports of an increased likelihood of moving from overweight to having obesity [70]. This relationship of weight stigma to increasing energy intake and thus weight should not be underestimated. It should inform practice and the use of language by all professions who come into contact with people of any age living with obesity and their families. This topic is returned to in later chapters.

Weight stigma in CYP has been reported to be associated with:

- Increased risk of depression
- Anxiety
- Social isolation
- Substance misuse
- Suicidal thoughts
- Poor body image
- Low self-esteem
- Unhealthy eating behaviours
- Decreased physical activity
- Increased weight gain [70, 72].

Studies over the years have shown that the problem of stigma is not new nor is it reducing but is becoming more prevalent. Latner and Stunkard reported that stigmatisation of children living with obesity was worse in a 2001 study compared to a similar study carried out in the 1960s [73]. Schwimmer et al. using the Pediatric Quality of Life Inventory (PedsQL) questionnaire reported that CYP living with obesity had a worse quality of life than CYP undergoing cancer treatment [74]. However, what has improved is the awareness of the stigma and bias and the adverse effects it causes, with policy documents such as this one from the WHO helping to ensure an awareness can lead to changes in attitudes and behaviours – WeightBias.pdf (who.int) [71].

> **WHAT DOES THIS MEAN FOR PRACTICE?**
>
> At the end of each chapter, there is a final section giving a summary of the author's thoughts on the practical application of the thoughts and information they have shared. For Chapter 1, this would be for the reader to consider in their practice the importance and complexity of obesity through childhood and into adulthood while understanding the significance of the bio-psycho-social interactions. Supporting CYP living with obesity and their families should have priority in all health and social care and not be dismissed as a personal choice. All health and social care professionals have a duty to approach CYP living with obesity in a non-judgemental and compassionate manner.

References

1 Gillespie, J., Midmore, C., Hoeflich, J. et al. (2015). Parents as the start of the solution: a social marketing approach to understanding triggers and barriers to entering a childhood weight management service. *J. Hum. Nutr. Diet.* 28: 83–92. https://doi.org/10.1111/jhn.12237.

2 World Health Organization (2021). Fact sheet: obesity and overweight. https://www.who.int/news-room/fact-sheets/detail/obesity-and-overweight (accessed 24 March 2023).

3 Lobstein, T. and Jackson-Leach, R. (2016). Planning for the worst: estimates of obesity and comorbidities in school-age children in 2025. *Pediatr. Obes.* 11: 321–325. https://doi.org/10.1111/ijpo.12185.

4 Bentham, J., Di Cesare, M., Bilano, V. et al. (2017). Worldwide trends in body-mass index, underweight, overweight, and obesity from 1975 to 2016: a pooled analysis of 2416 population-based measurement studies in 128·9 million children, adolescents, and adults. *Lancet* 390: 2627–2642. https://doi.org/10.1016/S0140-6736(17)32129-3.

5 Hampl, S.E., Hassink, S.G., Skinner, A.C. et al. (2023). Clinical practice guideline for the evaluation and treatment of children and adolescents with obesity. *Pediatrics* 151: e2022060640. https://doi.org/10.1542/peds.2022-060640.

6 Public Health England (2020). Disparities in the risk and outcomes of COVID-19. https://www.gov.uk/government/publications/covid-19-review-of-disparities-in-risks-and-outcomes (accessed 18 March 2024).

7 WHO (2000). Obesity: Preventing and Managing the Global Epidemic. Report of a WHO Consultation, Switzerland.

8 Freedman, D.S., Serdula, M.K., Srinivasan, S.R. et al. (1999). Relation of circumferences and skinfold thicknesses to lipid and insulin concentrations in children and adolescents: the Bogalusa Heart Study. *Am. J. Clin. Nutr.* 69: 308–317. https://doi.org/10.1093/ajcn/69.2.308.

9 Yamashita, S., Nakamura, T., Shimomura, L. et al. (1996). Insulin resistance and body fat distribution: contribution of visceral fat accumulation to the development of insulin resistance and atherosclerosis. *Diabetes Care* 19: 287–291. https://doi.org/10.2337/diacare.19.3.287.

10 Stewart, L. (2010). Childhood obesity. *Medicine (Baltimore)* 39: 42–44. https://doi.org/10.1097/00017285-197405000-00003.

11 Han, J.C., Lawlor, D.A., and SYS, K. (2010). Childhood obesity – 2010: progress and challenges determinants and risk factors for childhood obesity. *Childhood* 375: 1737–1748. https://doi.org/10.1016/S0140-6736(10)60171-7.

12 Goran, M.I. and Gower, B.A. (1999). Relation between visceral fat and disease risk in children and adolescents. *Am. J. Clin. Nutr.* 70: 149S–156S.

13 NICE (2023). Overview | Obesity: identification, assessment and management | Guidance| NICE (accessed 18 March 2024).

14 Maynard, L.M., Wisemandle, W., Roche, A.F. et al. (2001). Childhood body composition in relation to body mass index. *Pediatrics* 107: 344 LP–350 LP. https://doi.org/10.1542/peds.107.2.344.

15 Jebb, S.A. and Prentice, A.M. (2002). Single definition of overweight and obesity should be used. *BMJ* 323: 999. https://doi.org/10.1136/bmj.323.7319.999.

16 Himes, J.H. and Dietz, W.H. (1994). Guidelines for overweight in adolescent preventive services: recommendations from an expert committee. *Am. J. Clin. Nutr.* 59: 307–316. https://doi.org/10.1093/ajcn/59.2.307.

17 Chinn, S. (2006). Definitions of childhood obesity: current practice. *Eur. J. Clin. Nutr.* 60: 1189–1194. https://doi.org/10.1038/sj.ejcn.1602436.

18 Reilly, J.J., Dorosty, A.R., and Emmett, P.M. (2000). Identification of the obese child: adequacy of the body mass index for clinical practice and epidemiology. *Int. J. Obes.* 24: 1623–1627. https://doi.org/10.1038/sj.ijo.0801436.

19 Altman, D.G. (1999). *Practical Statistics for Medical Research*. London, UK: Chapman and Hall.

20 Dorosty, A.R., Emmett, P.M., Cowin, S.I.S. et al. (2000). Factors associated with early adiposity rebound. *Pediatrics* 105: 1115 LP–1118 LP. https://doi.org/10.1542/peds.105.5.1115.

21 Wright, C.M. (2015). Defining and measuring childhood obesity. In: *Early Years Nutrition and Healthy Weight* (ed. L. Stewart and J. Thompson), 30–39. Wiley.

22 Barlow, S.E. (2007). Expert committee recommendations regarding the prevention, assessment, and treatment of child and adolescent overweight and obesity: summary report. *Pediatrics* 120: S164–S192. https://doi.org/10.1542/peds.2007-2329c.

23 SACN, RCPCH (2012). Position statement: consideration of issues around the use of BMI centile thresholds for defining underweight, overweight and obesity in children aged 2–18 years in the UK, pp. 1–15.

24 Daniels, S.R., Khoury, P., and Morrison, J. (2001). Utility of different measures of body fat distribution in children and adolescents. *Am. J. Epidemiol.* 152: 1179–1184. https://doi.org/10.1093/aje/152.12.1179.

25 McCarthy, H.D., Jarrett, K.V., and Crawley, H.F. (2001). The development of waist circumference percentiles in British children aged 5.0–16.9 y. *Eur. J. Clin. Nutr.* 55: 902–907. https://doi.org/10.1038/sj.ejcn.1601240.

26 Freedman, D.S., Srinivasan, S.R., Burke, G.L. et al. (1987). Relation of body fat distribution to hyperinsulinemia in children and adolescents: the Bogalusa Heart Study. *Am. J. Clin. Nutr.* 46: 403–410. https://doi.org/10.1093/ajcn/46.3.403.

27 Guntsche, Z., Guntsche, E.M., Saraví, F.D. et al. (2010). Umbilical waist-to-height ratio and trunk fat mass index (DXA) as markers of central adiposity and insulin resistance in Argentinean children with a family history of metabolic syndrome. *J. Pediatr. Endocrinol. Metab.* 23: 245–256. https://doi.org/10.1515/jpem.2010.23.3.245.

28 Maffeis, C., Banzato, C., and Talamini, G. (2008). Waist-to-height ratio, a useful index to identify high metabolic risk in overweight children. *J. Pediatr.* 152: 207–213. https://doi.org/10.1016/j.jpeds.2007.09.021.

29 Butland, B., Jebb, S., Kopelman, P. et al. (2007). Tackling obesities: future choices – project report. *Foresight* 162. https://doi.org/10.1002/hep.20263.

30 Comuzzie, A.G. (2002). The emerging pattern of the genetic contribution to human obesity. *Best Pract. Res. Clin. Endocrinol. Metab.* 16: 611–621. https://doi.org/10.1053/beem.2002.0224.

31 Barsh, G.S., Farooqi, I.S., and Rahilly, S.O. (2000). Genetics of body-weight regulation. *Nature* 404: 644–651.

32 Farooqi, I.S. and O'Rahilly, S. (2006). Genetics of obesity in humans. *Endocr. Rev.* 27: 710–718. https://doi.org/10.1210/er.2006-0040.

33 Farooqi, I.S., Keogh, J.M., Yeo, G.S.H. et al. (2003). Clinical spectrum of obesity and mutations in the melanocortin 4 receptor gene. *N. Engl. J. Med.* 348: 1085–1095. https://doi.org/10.1056/NEJMoa022050.

34 Drop, S., Farooqi, I.S., O'Rahilly, S. et al. (2006). Heterozygosity for a POMC – null mutation and increased obesity risk in humans. *Diabetes* 55: 2549–2553. https://doi.org/10.2337/db06-0214.

35 Lobstein, T., Baur, L., and Uauy, R. (2004). Obesity in children and young people: a crisis in public health. *Obes. Rev.* 5: 4–85. https://doi.org/10.1111/j.1467-789x.2004.00133.x.

36 Kelnar, C.J.H. (1992). Endocrine gland disorders. In: *Forfar adn Arneil's Textbook of Paediatrics* (ed. A.G.M. Campbell and N. McIntosh), 1085–1171. Edinburgh: Churchill Livingstone.

37 Viner, R. and Nicholls, D. (2005). Managing obesity in secondary care: a personal practice. *Arch. Dis. Child.* 90: 385–390. https://doi.org/10.1136/adc.2004.062224.

38 Jones, C.M., Merrick, M.T., and Houry, D.E. (2020). Identifying and preventing adverse childhood experiences: implications for clinical practice. *JAMA - J. Am. Med. Assoc.* 323: 25–26. https://doi.org/10.1001/jama.2019.18499.

39 Schroeder, K., Schuler, B.R., Kobulsky, J.M. et al. (2021). The association between adverse childhood experiences and childhood obesity: a systematic review. *Obes. Rev.* 22: https://doi.org/10.1111/obr.13204.

40 Gardner, R., Feely, A., Layte, R. et al. (2019). Adverse childhood experiences are associated with an increased risk of obesity in early adolescence: a population-based prospective cohort study. *Pediatr. Res.* 86: 522–528. https://doi.org/10.1038/s41390-019-0414-8.

41 Ebbiling, C.B., Pawluk, D., and Ludwig, D.S. (2012). Childhood obesity public-health crisis, common sense cure. *Lancet* 360: 473–482.

42 Freedman, D.S., Khan, L.K., Dietz, W.H. et al. (2001). Relationship of childhood obesity to coronary heart disease risk factors in adulthood: the Bogalusa Heart Study. *Pediatrics* 108: 712 LP–718 LP. https://doi.org/10.1542/peds.108.3.712.

43 Freedman, D.S., Mei, Z., Srinivasan, S.R. et al. (2007). Cardiovascular risk factors and excess adiposity among overweight children and adolescents: the Bogalusa Heart Study. *J. Pediatr.* 150: https://doi.org/10.1016/j.jpeds.2006.08.042.

44 Whitaker, R.C., Wright, J.A., Pepe, M.S. et al. (1997). Predicting obesity in young adulthood from childhood and parental obesity. *N. Engl. J. Med.* 337: 869–873. https://doi.org/10.1056/NEJM199709253371301.

45 Dietz, W.H. (1998). Childhood weight affects adult morbidity and mortality. *J. Nutr.* 128: 411S–414S. https://doi.org/10.1093/jn/128.2.411s.

46 Geserick, M., Vogel, M., Gausche, R. et al. (2018). Acceleration of BMI in early childhood and risk of sustained obesity. *N. Engl. J. Med.* 379: 1303–1312. https://doi.org/10.1056/nejmoa1803527.

47 Di Angelantonio, E., Bhupathiraju, S.N., Wormser, D. et al. (2016). Body-mass index and all-cause mortality: individual-participant-data meta-analysis of 239 prospective studies in four continents. *Lancet* 388: 776–786. https://doi.org/10.1016/S0140-6736(16)30175-1.

48 Dietz, W.H. and Nelson, A. (1999). Barriers to the treatment of childhood obesity: a call to action. *J. Pediatr.* 134: 535–536. https://doi.org/10.1016/S0022-3476(99)70235-0.

49 Reilly, J.J., Methven, E., Mcdowell, Z.C. et al. (2003). Health consequences of obesity health consequences of obesity. *JAMA* 748–752. https://doi.org/10.1136/adc.88.9.748.

50 Jones, K.L. (2006). The dilemma of the metabolic syndrome in children and adolescents: disease or distraction? *Pediatr. Diabetes* 7: 311–321. https://doi.org/10.1111/j.1399-5448.2006.00212.x.

51 Miranda, P.J., DeFronzo, R.A., Califf, R.M. et al. (2005). Metabolic syndrome: definition, pathophysiology, and mechanisms. *Am. Heart J.* 149: 33–45. https://doi.org/10.1016/j.ahj.2004.07.013.

52 American Diabetes Association (2000). Type 2 diabetes in children and adolescents. *Pediatrics* 105: 671–680. https://doi.org/10.1542/peds.105.3.671.

53 Dietz, W.H. (2001). Overweight and precursors of type 2 diabetes mellitus in children and adolescents. *J. Pediatr.* 138: 453–454. https://doi.org/10.1067/mpd.2001.113635.

54 Burrows, N.R., Gregg, E.W., Geiss, L.S. et al. (2002). Type 2 diabetes among North adolescents: an epidemiologic health perspective. *J. Pediatr.* 136: 664–672. https://doi.org/10.1067/mpd.2000.105141.

55 Reinehr, T. (2005). Clinical presentation of type 2 diabetes mellitus in children and adolescents. *Int. J. Obes.* 29: S105–S110. https://doi.org/10.1038/sj.ijo.0803065.

56 Royal College of Paediatrics and Child Health (2021). National Paediatric Diabetes Audit (NPDA) spotlight audit reports | RCPCH. Spotlight Report on Type 2 Diabetes 2021.pdf (accessed 18 March 2024).

57 Steinberger, J. and Daniels, S.R. (2003). Obesity, insulin resistance, diabetes, and cardiovascular risk in children: an American Heart Association scientific statement from the Atherosclerosis, Hypertension, and Obesity in the Young Committee (Council on Cardiovascular Disease in the Young) and the Diabetes Committee (Council on Nutrition, Physical Activity, and Metabolism). *Circulation* 107: 1448–1453. https://doi.org/10.1161/01.CIR.0000060923.07573.F2.

58 Viner, R.M., Segal, T.Y., Lichtarowicz-Krynska, F. et al. (2005). Prevalence of the insulin resistance syndrome in obesity. *Arch. Dis. Child.* 90: 10–14. https://doi.org/10.1136/adc.2003.036467.

59 Weiss, R., Dziura, J., Burgert, T. et al. (2004). Obesity and the metabolic syndrome in children and adolescents. *N. Engl. J. Med.* 350: 2362–2374.

60 Sinha, R., Fisch, G., Teague, B. et al. (2002). Prevalence of impaired glucose tolerance among children and adolescents with marked obesity. *N. Engl. J. Med.* 346: 802–810.

61 Hanas, R. (2007). *Type 1 Diabetes in Children, Adolescents, and Young Adults: How to Become an Expert on Your Own Diabetes.* Class Publications https://books.google.co.uk/books?id=2lyIu4_5r4IC (accessed 18 March 2024).

62 Farrell, G.C. and Larter, C.Z. (2006). Nonalcoholic fatty liver disease: from steatosis to cirrhosis. *Hepatology* 43: 99–112. https://doi.org/10.1002/hep.20973.

63 Patton, H.M., Sirlin, C., Behling, C. et al. (2006). Pediatric nonalcoholic fatty liver disease: a critical appraisal of current data and implications for future research. *J. Pediatr. Gastroenterol. Nutr.* 43 (4): 415–427.

64 Schwimmer, J.B., Deutsch, R., Kahen, T. et al. (2006). Prevalence of fatty liver in children and adolescents. *Pediatrics* 118: 1388 LP–1393 LP. https://doi.org/10.1542/peds.2006-1212.

65 NICE (2016). Assessment and management of non-alcoholic fatty liver disease. *Chronic Disease Management* https://doi.org/10.33591/sfp.48.1.u5.

66 Speiser, P.W., Rudolf, M.C.J., Anhalt, H. et al. (2005). Consensus statement: childhood obesity. *J. Clin. Endocrinol. Metab.* 90: 1871–1887. https://doi.org/10.1210/jc.2004-1389.

67 Puhl, R.M. and Brownell, K.D. (2006). Confronting and coping with weight stigma: an investigation of overweight and obese adults. *Obesity* 14: 1802–1815. https://doi.org/10.1038/oby.2006.208.

68 Kenney, E.L., Gortmaker, S.L., Davison, K.K. et al. (2015). The academic penalty for gaining weight: a longitudinal, change-in-change analysis of BMI and perceived academic ability in middle school students. *Int. J. Obes.* 39: 1408–1413. https://doi.org/10.1038/ijo.2015.88.

69 Viner, R.M. and Cole, T.J. (2005). Adult socioeconomic, educational, social, and psychological outcomes of childhood obesity: a national birth cohort study. *Br. Med. J.* 330: 1354–1357. https://doi.org/10.1136/bmj.38453.422049.E0.

70 Brown, A., Flint, S.W., and Batterham, R.L. (2022). Pervasiveness, impact and implications of weight stigma. *eClin. Med.* 47: 101408. https://doi.org/10.1016/j.eclinm.2022.101408.

71 World Health Organization (2017). Weight bias and obesity stigma: considerations for the WHO European Region. WHO-EURO-2017-5369-45134-64401-eng.pdf (accessed 18 March 2024).

72 Rankin, J., Matthews, L., Cobley, S. et al. (2016). Psychological consequences of childhood obesity: psychiatric comorbidity and prevention. *Adolesc. Health Med. Ther.* 7: 125–146. https://doi.org/10.2147/AHMT.S101631.

73 Shrewsbury, V. and Wardle, J. (2008). Socioeconomic status and adiposity in childhood: a systematic review of cross-sectional studies 1990–2005. *Obesity* 16: 275–284. https://doi.org/10.1038/oby.2007.35.

74 Schwimmer, J.B., Burwinkle, T.M., and Varni, J.W. (2003). Health-related quality of life of severely obese children and adolescents. *JAMA* 289: 1813–1819. https://doi.org/10.1001/jama.289.14.1813.

2 Socio-Economic Inequalities and Childhood Obesity

Laura Stewart

'It's so multi-factorial, it's so not down to individual choice, it's so wrapped up into politics and social norms and beliefs and values'. [1]

Introduction

It is well documented that inequalities in socio-economic status (SES) have a negative impact on health and well-being. The 2008 WHO report on health equity described at least 200 million children worldwide as not meeting their full development potential due to inequalities. While noting early childhood as a period of enormous influence on the subsequent risk of obesity, malnutrition, heart disease and mental health difficulties [2]. Therefore, starting life and early years with the long-term adverse effect of health inequalities is a hindrance to lifelong physical and mental health, including, as this chapter will explore, a healthier weight.

The reason a chapter in a book on childhood weight management is being devoted to this topic is that it is well recognised in developed countries that there is a higher prevalence of childhood obesity in children living in lower SES groups. Readers should be aware, however, that the converse is reported in developing countries, that is a higher prevalence of obesity is seen in the wealthier parts of the population across all age groups. This continues to be seen until that country appears to reach an economical tipping point and then the inverse relationship between SES and childhood obesity prevalence, mirroring high income countries, starts to emerge [3–7]. This makes our knowledge and understanding of the relationship between SES and obesity in children, as well as their parents, an important issue for us to try and understand. Particularly in considering the ramifications depending on whether we work in a

Child and Adolescent Obesity: A Practical Approach to Clinical Weight Management,
First Edition. Edited by Laura Stewart.
© 2024 John Wiley & Sons Ltd. Published 2024 by John Wiley & Sons Ltd.

developed or developing countries, or indeed one which is in transition and beginning to show an increasing prevalence of obesity in adults and children in lower SES.

Health Inequalities

Health inequalities are seen across the world, even in countries considered to be developed and wealthy. Taking the UK as an example, the 1980 Black Report illuminated the issue of health inequalities between differing levels of SES, and raised the issue of health inequalities in childhood [8]. Thirty years later, the 2010 Marmot Report on 'Health Inequalities in England' highlighted the impact on health, mortality and the length of time spent in poor health between those in the lower compared to those in higher SES groups [5].

When discussing the issue of health inequalities terms such as deprivation or poverty are often used, the preferred term in this chapter and throughout this book is to discuss lower and higher SES. There are numerous methods to evaluate and describe SES. In the many reviews and papers discussed in this chapter, a wide range of tools have been used, mainly:

- Educational attainment level of the mother and/or the father
- Income of parent/s or family or household
- Occupation of the mother and/or the father
- Scores using multiple indices for example Townsend Score [9], Scottish Indices of Multiple Deprivation (SIMD) [10], Indices of Multiple Deprivation (IMD) [11], Socio-Economic Indexes for Areas (SEIFA) [12].

There have been a number of calls over many years to have a consistent approach in the method utilised to define SES in relation to nutrition and obesity research but to date there is no agreed consistent methodology. It may be helpful to consider the methods and measurements used in the particular country and institution of the reader.

Marmot 2010, and in the 2020 follow-up report, emphasised the fact that health inequalities are actually the result of social and economic inequalities within a society [5, 13]. He surmises that the inequitable social gradients cannot be totally removed from a society. However, both reports advocate that social justice should look to a levelling upwards and that this can be achieved through *proportionate universalism*, i.e. at a level seen as proportionate to the need. Both the 2010 and 2020 reports noted that the single most important recommendation is *to give every child the best start in life* [5, 13]. A philosophy that should, indeed, be embedded within all practitioners and underpinning all services in the field of childhood weight management.

Talking about the consequences of ill health and SES inequalities, Marmot 2010 showed that in England people living in the lowest SES neighbourhoods have a life expectancy seven years shorter than those living in the higher SES areas. Considered as an even more important fact is the number of years actually spent in ill health and with a consequent disability, with the difference in years free from disability between the lower and higher SES groups, in England, being 17 years. In a person living with obesity, this may manifest as difficulty in everyday living tasks, for example due to breathing and orthopaedic problems.

Many research papers and reports will discuss QALYS – Quality Adjusted Life Years [14]; this is primarily a health economic term which assumes to take into account both life length expected and the quality of the life lived. With obesity often being discussed as a 'gateway disease' to many of the morbidities which lead to ongoing long-term ill health and disability, such as CVD and type 2 diabetes, this is an important consideration for weight management practitioners, service managers and policymakers.

Marmot is explicit in describing the determinants of health and well-being inequalities being rooted in social and economic inequalities. With social position influencing the interacting factors of:

- Material circumstances
- Social environment
- Psychological factors
- Behavioural factors [5].

The report considers that a life course viewpoint is essential in tackling the health and social inequalities as well as a whole system approach involving communities and individuals [5, 13]. *'Create an enabling society that maximises individuals and community potential',* Marmot 2020 [13]. Whole system approaches in the terms of childhood weight and obesity are looked at in detail in Chapter 3. Many of the broad aspects of health and social inequalities discussed by Marmot can be applied to other developed countries across the world.

Malnutrition is often associated with lower SES and health inequalities. In 2020 the WHO revised its definition of malnutrition to accentuate what is commonly known as the double burden of malnutrition: Stating:

> *'Malnutrition, in all its forms, includes undernutrition (wasting, stunting, underweight), inadequate vitamins or minerals, overweight, obesity, and resulting diet-related noncommunicable diseases'* [15].

It is important for practitioners and policymakers to recognise that overweight and obesity are a manifestation of malnutrition (*bad* nutrition) and that a higher weight can mask an inadequate intake of important vitamins and minerals. This definition of malnutrition will be used as a standard through this book.

SES and Obesity

The Granddaddy of modern systematic reviews looking at the prevalence of obesity and SES is by Sobal and Stunkard, published in 1989. This review looked at 144 studies, published between 1933 and 1988, across the world in developed and developing countries [16]. The authors' headline finding was a strong inverse relationship between SES and obesity among women in developed countries, i.e. more obesity was seen in women living in lower SES. This inverse association was strong across all racial backgrounds. Their 1989 review found no consistent association for men or children in developed countries. While in developing countries their review found a strong positive relationship for SES and obesity in women, men and children, i.e. a higher prevalence of obesity in populations living in higher SES [16].

In their review, Sobal and Stunkard found little agreement on the preferred measurement/s for SES, with the most commonly used ones being income, education level and occupation. With most studies they reviewed using only one measurement, they recommended that future studies used multiple measures of SES. Unsurprisingly, for children the SES of their parents or family were used as an indicator, with the SES of parents being the best indicator of the future SES of their children. While having parents living with obesity was one of the best predictors of their children having obesity [16]. Subsequent studies have found that parental education as an indicator of SES has a particular inverse relationship with child obesity, i.e. parents living in lower SES, as measured by educational attainment, have a higher prevalence of children with obesity [17–19].

In more recent work, Miyawaki et al. reported, in Organisation for Economic Cooperation and Development (OECD) countries, an inverse association between the amount of public social money spent on CYP and the prevalence of childhood obesity in that society. The important aspects of spending noted by the authors were on both early years education and care and school education [20].

Bentley et al. looked at the evolving inverse relationship of household income between obesity and type 2 diabetes in the US [21]. The authors noted that using US annual income, obesity and type 2 diabetes prevalence statistics, the inverse relationship can be seen to develop in the US from 1990 to a strong correlation by 2015. They state that in 1990 the typical prevalence figures for obesity in States across the US was 11% and by 2015 the obesity prevalence in all States was 20% or above, with the prevalence in several States above 35%. These authors made the interesting comment that from a genetic and human phenotype perspective, this shift in the prevalence of obesity in developed countries should be viewed as unprecedented [21].

SES and Obesity in Childhood

As mentioned earlier, there is now robust and undeniable evidence that there is a strong association between children living in a lower SES and having obesity in developed countries [3]. With this being a shift appearing since the 1989 Sobal and Stunkard review [16]. In 2008, Shrewsbury and Wardle carried out a systematic review looking at SES and adiposity in children. They found that the inverse relationship with lower SES and childhood adiposity was seen to be emerging in developed countries by 2005. Whereas in developing countries they still saw the opposite of a strong positive association for all age groups and genders between higher SES and adiposity [22].

A cross-sectional study looking at the prevalence of both obesity and underweight in Scottish children aged 5 years old over time found a similar trend to that described by Bentley in the US [21, 23]. Stewart et al. noted that although the overall prevalence of childhood obesity in this age group in Scotland had only risen slightly between 2011/2012 and 2017/2018, during this same period there in fact was a widening of inequalities with those living in the most deprived areas having a greater risk of living with obesity by 2017/2018 [23]. As an example of this change in the demographic distribution of high BMI with a higher prevalence in those in low SES within a developed country, see Figure 2.1. This graph shows the BMI distribution as measured across Scotland in the school years 2001/2002 to 2018/2019 [25]. This visual representation demonstrates clearly that while the overall figures show a consistently stable prevalence rate, there has been a growing and obvious difference in the prevalence in the population when drilled down to looked at by SES, in this case using SIMD. It is worth noting that a UK report on type 2 diabetes in CYP, the vast majority living with obesity at diagnosis, of these 71.4% lived in the lower SES and 65.1% were of a minority ethnic background [26].

While Australian studies looking at the prevalence of overweight and obesity in CYP from indigenous backgrounds as being 50% more likely to have overweight or obesity than non-indigenous CYP. Noting that living in a lower SES and coming from an indigenous background as being the *clearest independent predictors* of developing overweight and obesity [27]. In the US, studies show that racial and ethnic minority

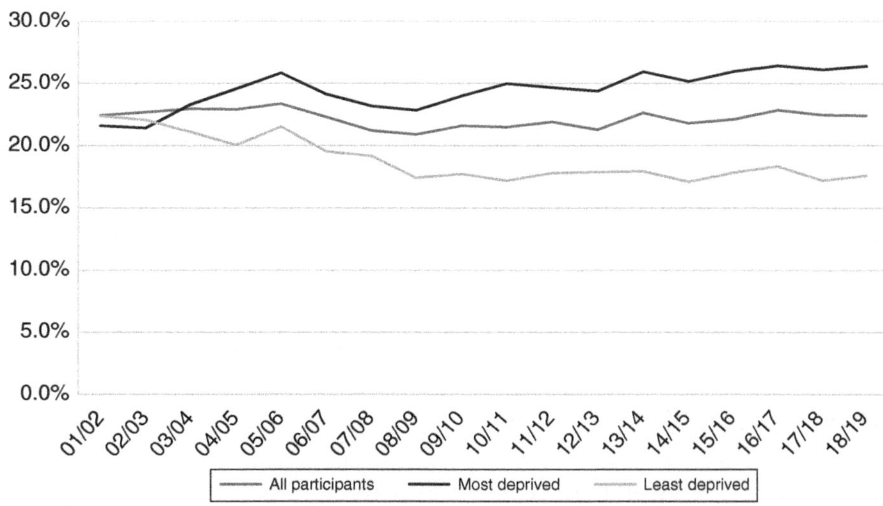

Figure 2.1 BMI distribution[a] of children across Scotland school years 2001/2002–2018/2019 by SES[b]. [a]BMI shown is ≥85th centile; using epidemiological cut-off points of 85th centile as at risk of overweight and 95th centile as at risk of obesity (WHO/UK 1990 charts) [24]. [b]Deprivation derived from SMID quintiles: 1, most deprived; 5, least deprived [9].

children (Hispanic and African American) from low SES have a higher prevalence of living with overweight and obesity [28, 29].

Influence of Parental Weight on Children

One of the reasons we discuss adult weight here and why it is important in the context of childhood obesity is the association between parents and their children's body weight. Whitaker et al., in an important 2010 paper, noted that *'there is a strong and graded association between parental weight status and risk of childhood obesity, which is significantly stronger for maternal weight'* [30]. A 2012 family cohort study over three generations found a positive correlation between maternal grandmother, mother and child with higher weight levels [31].

Consistently systematic reviews note that in the wealthier, developed countries the woman who are described as having a lower income, being less educated and less food secure are often more likely to live with overweight or obesity [6, 7, 16, 32, 33]. Indeed, in their 1989 review Sobal and Stunkard [16] discussed what they described as the first empirical study on this relationship, published in the 1960s, which established that the prevalence of obesity was six times higher in woman in lower compared to higher SES groups [34]. This demonstrates that the reverse SES – obesity relationship seen in women has been present in the US for a number of generations.

Keane et al. in 2012, while looking at paternal weight status, familial SES and childhood obesity at age 9 in a cohort taking part in 'Growing Up in Ireland' found an inverse association between maternal education level and child obesity. Describing maternal education as the most consistent SES indicator being associated with child obesity [17]. On the other hand, a 2017 systematic review by Wang et al., while agreeing with the association between parental and child overweight or obesity status, did not find a stronger association between mothers than fathers and child obesity [35].

Parental influences on early feeding and eating habits are cited as a factor in developing less healthy lifestyle and eating behaviours in families from lower SES. For example:

- Using formula milk in first six months
- The early introduction of solids
- Babies going to bed with a bottle of milk [27].

The education attainment level of the parents, talked about above as negatively associated with child obesity, is considered by some to be a possible factor in the difficulties to communicate effective public health messages [18]. Zhang et al. 2021 found that the least healthy lifestyles with highest risks of mortality and CVD were seen in adults in lower SES groups [36]. Targeted public health messaging will be returned to in Chapter 3 on whole systems approaches.

Food Insecurity

The underlying reasons for this inverse association between SES and childhood obesity in developed countries are numerous and complex [37]. It is easier to comprehend the positive correlation between higher SES and obesity prevalence in adults and children seen in developing countries. Where those with the higher level of income can afford both the quantities of food and the breadth of food types including those higher in energy that leads to a habitual intake of higher energy than body requirements. While those living in lower SES struggle to have enough money to buy the food to buy their daily energy requirements. A group living in high income countries but often suffering from food insecurities and nutritional inadequacies are international refugees [38], a group to be kept in mind when considering the issues discussed in this and other chapters.

The need for using food banks is a potent indictor of families and individuals struggling with food insecurity. Food banks provide food parcels to people living on low incomes and in situations where they cannot afford to purchase these themselves. A typical food parcel could include – breakfast cereal, soup, pasta, rice, tinned vegetables and sauces, lentils, beans, pulses, tinned meat, tea/coffee, tinned fruit, biscuits, UHT milk, fruit juice and often essential non-food items like toiletries and hygiene products [39].

The Trussell Trust (`www.trusselltrust.org`) in the UK has commissioned on-going research looking into the need and the use of UK food banks. Around 700,000 households (2.5% of all UK households) used a food bank in 2019/2020. With the COVID-19 lockdowns impacting on these numbers with a 46% increase in the number of CYP supported by the Trussell Trust food banks from 2018/2019 to 2019/2020 [40].

This leads us to discuss food insecurity in developed countries and what some call the poverty-obesity paradox. Keenan et al. define food insecurity as *'unreliable access to nutritionally adequate and safe foods'* [41]. These authors note that Franklin et al. in 2012 reported that food insecurity has been found to be a robust predictor of both adult and childhood obesity [41, 42]. Hruschka calls this the poverty-obesity paradox. This being when living in enduring deprivation leads to food choices that are less expensive but *paradoxically* tend to have a higher energy content. Particularly in Western, developed countries there is wide spread use of processed, inexpensive, predominately high-energy 'junk' foods [21]. Keenan has noted that household food insecurity is directly associated with poorer diet quality [41].

These higher energy foods often contain low nutrient value and can encourage overconsumption. The long-term intake of these low-nutrient, high-energy food products combined with a lifestyle of low levels of physical activities lead to long-term weight gain resulting in developing overweight and obesity [6].

Food insecurity has been described as being strongly associated with anxiety, depression and emotional distress. While in turn, emotional distress has been found to be associated with increased food intake and obesity [43, 44]. Bentley et al. talk about those living in deprivation receiving more cues derived from the stress of their daily lives which encourage the eating of less expensive, more processed foods including sugar-sweetened drinks [21]. One study reported by Keenan et al. showed no direct association between distress and obesity [41]. However, what these authors and others do discuss is one coping mechanism for distress recognised as increased eating, including taking larger portion sizes, binge eating behaviours and increased consumption of alcohol, which all in turn can adversely affect weight [3, 41].

The role of polygenetics in the development of obesity has been touched on in Chapter 1. While without a doubt genetics play a role in making some people more susceptible to weight and adipose gain, it cannot explain the modern rise in the prevalence of obesity and particularly extreme obesity [45]. Therefore, work has looked at environment and cultural drivers of obesity as well as the underlying biological ones. This has led to the emergence of a number of hypotheses and theoretical models which attempt to explain why humans (and often other mammals and birds) store body fat and are thus prone to obesity. These include but are not limited to:

- The insurance hypothesis [7]
- FTO gene [46]
- The thrifty gene hypothesis [47, 48]
- Modern environment leading to decreased energy expenditure [49].

Insurance Hypothesis

The insurance hypothesis (IH), as elucidated by Nettle et al., is one such model hypothesis. IH tries to explain why the drive to store fat in the human body may be associated with lower SES and food insecurity. The IH is part of adaptive evolutionary thinking, that the human body is evolutionarily programmed to store body fat to act as a safeguard against periods of short fall in food provision. 'Cues' are received from the environment when individuals are in situations of insecurity/uncertainty of food provision. A cue of sustained reduced food availability drives an individual to store body fat as an insurance against long term food insecurity. Thereby, making food insecurity a proximate driver of eating more energy and increasing body weight [7]. Nettle et al. postulated that the IH partially helps to explain why income inequality and individual poverty increase the risk of high BMI in developed countries. However, since numerous studies across many developed countries demonstrate this more strongly in woman than men the IH cannot fully explain all the complex drivers of modern obesity [7].

The Neighbourhood and Built Environment

The neighbourhood people live in, particularly the built environment of the neighbourhood, is another aspect often mooted of why those living in lower SES environments are more prone in finding making healthier lifestyle choices difficult [18, 28]. Consider that in certain neighbourhoods there may be fewer opportunities to use organised leisure facilities or that any such nearby facilities are outside of the budget that families can afford, therefore not being a priority. Taking walks or playing outside may feel unsafe. It has been demonstrated that in a neighbourhood with high levels of crime there is a link to lower levels of physical activity and thus energy output [28]. There can be no doubt that parents will put their children's safety before the use of outside space for physical activity and play.

In the neighbourhood there may be limited shopping facilities for choice of healthier foods at reasonable prices. For example, access to less healthier foods (energy dense such as those that are high in fat, sugar and salt but low in essential macro and micronutrients – see Chapter 7) has increased since the advent of the obesity epidemic. These less healthier/ higher energy foods are often on promotion in supermarkets and other local food outlets using lower pricing schemes and what is colloquially called a 'buy one get one free' (BOGOF) offers. It is unsurprising that in a family situation where money is tight that these become the preferred option when purchasing the family food and drink. There is also evidence to suggest that CYP are more likely to have overweight or obesity if there are fast food outlets near their home or school.

It should come as no surprise that parents and their families are less able to adopt healthier lifestyles, around both physical activity and food choices, unless positive changes to their economic, physical and social environment can be made. In practical terms, this requires local and national governments to create and fund policies to help communities to enhance their built environment to, in turn, promote and improve healthier lifestyles choices. A whole systems approach (WSA) is a concept that has arisen out of this type of thinking. It looks at local approaches, relying on community engagement and utilising 'local assets'. The WSA is an important emerging field around childhood obesity prevention and is explored in depth in Chapter 3.

WHAT DOES THIS MEAN FOR PRACTICE?

This is without doubt a complex issue, involving societal, economic and health interactions. For those living in affluent, westernised, developed countries, you will come across the phenomena of a higher prevalence of obesity in women and children living in lower SES. While for those working in developing countries, a higher prevalence of obesity for adults and children will be seen in those living in the higher SES of society. In some societies, it is an upwards challenge to change societal perceptions such as overweight and obesity being seen as a sign of wealth and good fortune.

In developed countries, the poverty-obesity paradox means putting thought and energy into considering how best to target and engage with those living in lower SES. Both childhood obesity treatment and prevention strategies require to take this into consideration. The Lobstein et al. review looking at social disparities in treatment for children aged 3–10 years found poor quality evidence on specific treatment approaches at differing SES context [50]. For the most part work to tackle social and economic inequalities are beyond the scope of the role of those working in weight management other than to be advocates for social, economic and health change. National and local government planning and policies need to be in place and action to make an in-road to changing overall inequalities and health inequalities.

Taking a whole systems approach (see Chapter 3) working at a neighbourhood or ward level can help to gather the right information on what matters to the people living in the area and how best to work with them on realising meaningful change. The National Institute for Clinical Excellence (NICE) in England recommend that any clinical service be appropriate to the culture of the group it is serving [51, 52]. This includes materials advertising the service, location of the service and programme materials, as well as ethnic background partitioners should consider these in light of SES background.

Thought needs to be given to ease of access to clinical sessions (whether groups or one to one) with regular inexpensive public transport. While programme reading materials require to be of a suitable educational level for both the CYP and adults taking part.

References

1 Stewart, L. (2021). Personal communication: practitioner.
2 World Health Organization (2008). Closing the gap in a generation: health equity through action on the social determinants of health. https://www.who.int/publications/i/item/WHO-IER-CSDH-08.1 (accessed 29 March 2024).
3 El-Sayed, A.M., Scarborough, P., and Galea, S. (2012). Socioeconomic inequalities in childhood obesity in the United Kingdom: a systematic review of the literature. *Obes. Facts* 5: 671–692. https://doi.org/10.1159/000343611.
4 Kim, Y., Cubbin, C., and Oh, S. (2019). A systematic review of neighbourhood economic context on child obesity and obesity-related behaviours. *Obes. Rev.* 20: 420–431. https://doi.org/10.1111/obr.12792.
5 Marmot, M. (2010). Strategic Review of Health Inequalities in England Post-2010. Fair-Society-Healthy-Lives-Full-Marmot Report 2010. https://www.gov.uk/research-for-development-outputs/fair-society-healthy-lives-the-marmot-review-strategic-review-of-health-inequalities-in-england-post-2010 (accessed 29 March 2024).
6 Hruschka, D.J. (2012). Do economic constraints on food choice make people fat? A critical review of two hypotheses for the poverty-obesity paradox. *Am. J. Hum. Biol.* 24: 277–285. https://doi.org/10.1002/ajhb.22231.
7 Nettle, D., Andrews, C., and Bateson, M. (2017). Food insecurity as a driver of obesity in humans: the insurance hypothesis. *Behav. Brain Sci.* 40: 1–53. https://doi.org/10.1017/S0140525X16000947.

8   Department of Health and Social Security (1980). Inequalities in Health: Report of a Research Working Group (The Black Report), London, UK.

9   Townsend, P., Phillimore, P., and Beattie, A. (1988). *Health and Deprivation: Inequalities and the North*. London, UK: Routledge.

10 Scottish Government (2020). Scottish Indices of Multiple Deprivation (SIMD). https://www.gov.scot/news/scottish-index-of-multiple-deprivation-2020/ (accessed 9 April 2021).

11 GOV.UK (2019). English Indices of Multiple Deprivation (IMD). https://www.gov.uk/guidance/english-indices-of-deprivation-2019-mapping-resources (accessed 9 April 2021).

12 Australian Bureau of Statistics (2016). Socio-Economic Indexes for Areas (SEIFA). https://www.abs.gov.au/ausstats/abs@.nsf/mf/2033.0.55.001 (accessed 9 April 2021).

13 Institiute of Health Equity (2020). Health equity in England: the marmot review 10 years on. https://www.health.org.uk/publications/reports/the-marmot-review-10-years-on (accessed 29 May 2024).

14 Howren, M.B. (2013). Quality-adjusted life years (QALYs). In: *Encyclopedia of Behavioral Medicine* (ed. M.D. Gellman and J.R. Turner). New York, NY: Springer https://doi.org/10.1007/978-1-4419-1005-9_613.

15 WHO (2020). Malnutrition: fact sheet. https://www.who.int/news-room/fact-sheets/detail/malnutrition (accessed 23 March 2021).

16 Sobal, J. and Stunkard, A.J. (1989). Socioeconomic status and obesity: a review of the literature. *Psychol. Bull.* 105: 260–275. https://doi.org/10.1037/0033-2909.105.2.260.

17 Keane, E., Layte, R., Harrington, J. et al. (2012). Measured parental weight status and familial socio-economic status correlates with childhood overweight and obesity at age 9. *PLoS One* 7. https://doi.org/10.1371/journal.pone.0043503.

18 Barriuso, L., Miqueleiz, E., Albaladejo, R. et al. (2015). Socioeconomic position and childhoodadolescent weight status in rich countries: a systematic review, 1990–2013. *BMC Pediatr.* 15: 1–15. https://doi.org/10.1186/s12887-015-0443-3.

19 Hampl, S.E., Hassink, S.G., Skinner, A.C. et al. (2023). Clinical practice guideline for the evaluation and treatment of children and adolescents with obesity. *Pediatrics* 151: e2022060640. https://doi.org/10.1542/peds.2022-060640.

20 Miyawaki, A., Evans, C.E.L., Lucas, P.J. et al. (2021). Relationships between social spending and childhood obesity in OECD countries: an ecological study. *BMJ Open* 11: e044205. https://doi.org/10.1136/bmjopen-2020-044205.

21 Bentley, R.A., Ormerod, P., and Ruck, D.J. (2018). Recent origin and evolution of obesity-income correlation across the United States. *Palgrave Commun.* 4: 1–14. https://doi.org/10.1057/s41599-018-0201-x.

22 Shrewsbury, V. and Wardle, J. (2008). Socioeconomic status and adiposity in childhood: a systematic review of cross-sectional studies 1990–2005. *Obesity* 16: 275–284. https://doi.org/10.1038/oby.2007.35.

23 Stewart, R., Reilly, J.J., Hughes, A. et al. (2021). Trends in socioeconomic inequalities in underweight and obesity in 5-year-old children, 2011–2018: population-based, repeated cross – sectional study. *BMJ Open* 11. https://doi.org/10.1136/bmjopen-2020-042023.

24 The Scottish Government (2020). The Scottish Health Survey 2019 Edition: Main Report. http://doi.org/10.4135/9781446273 05013501440

25 ISD Scotland (2019). Body mass index of primary 1 children in Scotland: school year 2018/19. https://www.statisticsauthority.gov.uk/national-statistician/types-of-official-statistics/ (accessed 25 September 2020).

26 Royal College of Paediatrics and Child Health (2021). NPDA spotlight audit report type 2 diabetes. www.rcpch.ac.uk/sites/default/files/2021-11/NPDA. Spotlight Report on Type 2 Diabetes 2021.pdf (accessed 13 April 2023).

27 Laws, R., Campbell, K.J., Van Der Pligt, P. et al. (2014). The impact of interventions to prevent obesity or improve obesity related behaviours in children (0-5 years) from socioeconomically disadvantaged and/or indigenous families: a systematic review. *BMC Publ. Health* 14: https://doi.org/10.1186/1471-2458-14-779.

28 Johnson, K.A., Showell, N.N., Flessa, S. et al. (2019). Do neighborhoods matter? A systematic review of modifiable risk factors for obesity among low socio-economic status black and hispanic children. *Child. Obes.* 15: 71–86. https://doi.org/10.1089/chi.2018.0044.

29 Nobari, T.Z., Whaley, S.E., Prelip, M.L. et al. (2018). Trends in socioeconomic disparities in obesity prevalence among low-income children aged 2–4 years in Los Angeles County, 2003–2014. *Child. Obes.* 14: 248–258. https://doi.org/10.1089/chi.2017.0264.

30 Whitaker, K.L., Jarvis, M.J., Beeken, R.J. et al. (2010). Comparing maternal and paternal intergenerational transmission of obesity. *Am. J. Clin. Nutr.* 91: 1560–1567. https://doi.org/10.3945/ajcn.2009.28838.1560.

31 Murrin, C.M., Kelly, G.E., Tremblay, R.E. et al. (2012). Body mass index and height over three generations: evidence from the Lifeways cross-generational cohort study. *BMC Publ. Health* 12: 81. https://doi.org/10.1186/1471-2458-12-81.

32 Newton, S., Braithwaite, D., and Akinyemiju, T.F. (2017). Socio-economic status over the life course and obesity: systematic review and meta-analysis. *PLoS One* 5: 1–15. https://doi.org/10.1371/journal.pone.0177151.

33 Cohen, A.K., Rai, M., Rehkopf, D.H. et al. (2013). Educational attainment and obesity: a systematic review. *Obes. Rev.* 14: 989–1005. https://doi.org/10.1111/obr.12062.

34 Goldblatt, P.B., Moore, M.E., and Stunkard, A.J. (1965). Social factors in obesity. *JAMA* 192: 1039–1044. https://doi.org/10.1001/jama.1965.03080250017004.

35 Wang, Y., Min, J., Khuri, J. et al. (2017). A systematic examination of the association between parental and child obesity across countries. *Adv. Nutr.* 8: 436–448. https://doi.org/10.3945/an.116.013235.

36 Zhang, Y.-B., Chen, C., Pan, X.-F. et al. (2021). Associations of healthy lifestyle and socioeconomic status with mortality and incident cardiovascular disease: two prospective cohort studies. *BMJ* 372: n604. https://doi.org/10.1136/bmj.n604.

37 Butland B, Jebb S, Kopelman P, et al. Tackling Obesities: Future Choices – Project Report. Foresight. https://www.semanticscholar.org/paper/Foresight.-Tackling-obesities:-future-choices.-Butland-Jebb/e7fb5766dc0838ea5e 163218214f65994ab4599f (accessed 29 May 2024).

38 Mansour, R., Liamputtong, P., and Arora, A. (2020). Prevalence, determinants, and effects of food insecurity among middle eastern and north african migrants and refugees in high-income countries: a systematic review. *Int. J. Environ. Res. Publ. Health* 17: 1–19. https://doi.org/10.3390/ijerph17197262.

39 Trussell Trust (2023). Emergency food parcels. www.trusselltrust.org/get-help/emergency-food/food-parcel/ (accessed 12 April 2023).

40 Bramley G, Treanor M, Sosenko F, et al. (2021). State of hunger: building the evidence on poverty, AQAQAQ, and food insecurity in the UK. www.trusselltrust.org/wp-content/uploads/sites/2/2021/05/State-of-Hunger-2021-Report-Final.pdf (accessed 29 May 2024).

41 Keenan, G.S., Christiansen, P., and Hardman, C.A. (2021). Household food insecurity, diet quality, and obesity: an explanatory model. *Obesity* 29: 143–149. https://doi.org/10.1002/oby.23033.

42 Franklin, B., Jones, A., Love, D. et al. (2012). Exploring mediators of food insecurity and obesity: a review of recent literature. *J. Community Health* 37: 253–264. https://doi.org/10.1007/s10900-011-9420-4.

43 Gibson, E.L. (2012). The psychobiology of comfort eating: implications for neuropharmacological interventions. *Behav. Pharmacol.* 23: 442–460. https://doi.org/10.1097/FBP.0b013e328357bd4e.

44 Laitinen, J., Ek, E., and Sovio, U. (2002). Stress-related eating and drinking behavior and body mass index and predictors of this behavior. *Prev. Med. (Baltim.)* 34: 29–39. https://doi.org/10.1006/pmed.2001.0948.

45 Qasim, A., Turcotte, M., de Souza, R.J. et al. (2018). On the origin of obesity: identifying the biological, environmental and cultural drivers of genetic risk among human populations. *Obes. Rev.* 19: 121–149. https://doi.org/10.1111/obr.12625.

46 Frayling, T.M., Timpson, N.J., Weedon, M.N. et al. (2007). Index and predisposes to childhood and adult obesity. *Science (80-)* 316: 889–894. https://doi.org/10.1126/science.1141634.A.

47 Prentice, A.M. (2001). Fires of life: the struggles of an ancient metabolism in a modern world. *Nutr. Bull.* 26: 13–27. https://doi.org/10.1046/j.1467-3010.2001.00100.x.

48 Neel, J.V. (1962). Diabetes mellitus: a 'thrifty' genotype rendered detrimental by 'progress'? *Am. J. Hum. Genet.* 14: 353–362.

49 Prentice, A.M. and Jebb, S.A. (1995). Obesity in Britain: gluttony or sloth? *BMJ Br. Med. J.* 311: 437. https://doi.org/10.1136/bmj.311.7002.437.

50 Lobstein, T., Neveux, M., Brown, T. et al. (2021). Social disparities in obesity treatment for children age 3–10 years: a systematic review. *Obes. Rev.* 22: 1–13. https://doi.org/10.1111/obr.13153.

51 NICE (2014). Obesity: identification, assessment and management of overweight and obesity in children young people and adults CG189. `https://www.nice.org.uk/guidance/cg189` (accessed 29 May 2024).
52 NICE (2013). Managing overweight and obesity among children and young people: lifestyle weight management services PH47. `https://www.nice.org.uk/guidance/cg189` (accessed 29 May 2024).

3 Systems Thinking and Systems Approaches to Address Obesity

Jenny Gillespie

'Particularly for such a complex topic like this where there is no one organisation that has sole responsibility for this, nor does it have all the solutions'. [1]

Introduction

No country's Government has managed to reverse the rising tide of obesity prevalence in children or adults over the last three decades, despite numerous plans and strategies that have attempted to address the issue. Understanding more about this 'policy inertia' and what has been unsuccessful in the past is important for future learning and improvement. In 2013, a paper that presented progress in obesity prevention in Australia and New Zealand over a 20-year period concluded that despite multiple reports, strong advocacy, and good examples of community-level action, key fiscal, public sector and regulatory policies were largely unimplemented due to private sector and lobbying pressure being embedded within public policy development [2]. Almost a decade later an analysis of over 700 obesity strategies and policies in England between 1992 and 2020 highlighted that the way in which these strategies and policies are proposed reduces the likelihood of them being implemented. It concluded that attempts to address the issue of obesity have failed in part because of the repetition of very similar policies, lessons not being learned from one government plan to the next and because the many policies have been consistently weak in their design, implementation and/or evaluation [3].

It is widely recognised that obesity is a complex and multifactorial disease with root causes that include, among others, biological or genetic

Child and Adolescent Obesity: A Practical Approach to Clinical Weight Management, First Edition. Edited by Laura Stewart.

factors and the interaction between individuals, families or communities with the food and/or the built ('obesogenic') environment and commercial determinants that surround us. The UK Foresight Report proposed that population levels of obesity are the result of a complex adaptive system and that systems thinking and systems approaches should be adopted when trying to navigate and alter such systems [4, 5].

The aims of this chapter are:

1. To outline **systems definitions and systems theory**, by describing key concepts of systems thinking and systems approaches as a means to account for the complexity of addressing obesity within the context of public health.
2. To provide examples of the **application** of systems approaches to obesity through implementation case studies from across the world.
3. To provide examples of the **evaluation systems approaches to obesity** in the real-world settings.
4. To put forward the **opportunities, challenges and future direction of systems approaches to obesity**

The practical illustrations will be particularly useful to practitioners and policymakers who work in the field of public health, obesity prevention and/or management.

Systems Definitions and Systems Theory

Lay Definitions

It is not easy to define a system, various descriptions exist and these are drawn from multiple theories, wide ranging perspectives and diverse disciplines. With origins in the field of mathematics and biology, in the early 20th century, systems theory was widely applied to a number of subjects, including computer science, sociology management, law, psychology and most recently to social sciences [6].

From the early 1970s to the late 1990s, the work of Donella Meadows, an influential American environmental thinker and scholar, helped define and understand the functioning of systems. Donella Meadows described a systems as *'a set of things – people, cells, molecules, or whatever – interconnected in such a way that they produce their own pattern of behaviour over time. The system may be buffeted, constricted, triggered, or driven by outside forces. But the system's response to these forces is characteristic of itself, and that response is seldom simple in the real world.'* Further adding that *'A system is more than the sum of its parts. It may exhibit adaptive, dynamic, goal-seeking, self-preserving, and sometimes evolutionary behaviour'* [7].

By the late 1990s, papers on systems change in the context of public services [8] and public health were beginning to appear in the literature by Meadows [7, 9, 10], Foster-Fishman [11, 12] and others.

One definition of a system offered by Foster-Fishman is: *'the set of actors, activities, and settings that are directly or indirectly perceived to have influence in or be affected by a given problem situation.'* And systems change described as *'An intentional process designed to alter the status quo by shifting and realigning the form and function of a targeted system'* [11].

In the Chronic Disease Prevention (CDP) policy landscape, the WHO has published a guidance manual in which it described systems thinking as a rapidly developing area of knowledge in CDP and defined systems thinking as follows: *'the process of considering the bigger picture when developing a solution to a problem. This style of thinking is especially important when trying to create solutions to complex problems that are influenced by a range of dynamic factors, including individuals, populations and organizations, all requiring consideration'.* Systems approaches are defined *as: 'methods or methodologies that encourage the implementation of systems thinking'* [13].

The manual is useful for policymakers as it outlines the application of a range of key concepts associated with systems thinking, shown in Table 3.1 [11].

Table 3.1 Key concepts in systems thinking.

Concept	Definition
Systems thinking	A set of ideas and methods which encourage us to look at the bigger picture
Systems approaches	Specific methods or methodologies (a set of procedures for gathering or interpreting data and/or evidence) informed by systems thinking principles.
Leverage point	A point in a system where a small intervention can lead to substantial, system-wide changes.
Unintended consequence	Response provoked when intervening in a system that is unintended or difficult to predict (can be harmful or beneficial)
Nonlinear relationship	A relationship between two elements in a system where the cause does not produce a proportional effect
Feedback loop	A closed chain of casual connections resulting in the output of a system or system element feeding back into itself
Delay	An interval of time between cause and effect, which can create instability and fluctuations in system behaviour.

Source: World Health Organization [14]/https://iris.who.int/bitstream/handle/10665/357174/WHO-EURO-2022-4195-43954-61946-eng.pdf?sequence=1/last accessed November 14, 2022.

Further expansion of each of the concepts outlined in Table 3.1 is available in the wider systems literature including some of those cited earlier in this chapter [7–12]. Though out with the scope of this chapter, the WHO manual also described a range of qualitative and quantitative system methods, e.g. causal loop diagram, system dynamic modelling and network analysis among others, that can further aid understanding of a system.

A 2019 systematic review by Australian authors sought to understand how systems are defined in the literature, to uncover key attributes, and describe how systems approaches are considered. No useful working definition for a system for CDP was found so authors formulated a working definition as follows: *'multiple entities and actions that work in dynamic ways to affect the complex array of factors that contribute to CDP'* where 'actions' are policies, programmes, interventions, strategies, approaches, projects, laws and regulations. They developed four themed elements that summarised how parts of the system were described and seven attributes of effective systems to create a framework to strengthen the practical application of systems for CDP [15].

Systems Theory

There is a perception that systems approaches are too difficult to apply, do not explicitly reference the systems way of thinking or have not been suitably designed or evaluated [16].

To overcome some of the challenges associated with operationalising systems approaches in Public Health, Foster-Fishman et al. published a seminal paper in 2007 [11]. Here, a range of systems theories and concepts from many fields were synthesised in order to address the 'concept gap' dilemma – that the reality of systems functioning, e.g. complex, interconnected parts, is at odds with the prevailing 'linear' thinking of those driving systems change efforts. Authors articulated that systems change is about shifting the status quo by altering the elemental form and functioning of a system, thus adopting any change also requires a shift in practices and behaviours by the system change agents. They went on to describe that system change effort are complex, challenging and require a suitable framework that accounts for the dynamics properties and nature of system that they are trying to change.

A crucial aspect of understanding the system is to analyse three key attributes of each system part:

1. its character within the system including how it is similar and different across different system actors and subsystems
2. the extent to which it coheres with the goals of the systems change endeavour

3. how it influences and is influenced by other fundamental parts while simultaneously considering the interactions with other system characteristics.

'A framework for systems change' was developed to support analysis of the three attributes, comprising of four 'principled steps':

1. bounding the system
2. understanding fundamental system parts as potential root causes (includes 'below the surface' and 'apparent level' elements and structures)
3. assessing the system interactions
4. identifying levers for change.

Additionally, a set of guiding questions assists in examining 5 key systems characteristics.

Foster-Fishman et al., subsequently put forward the 'Above and Below Line' (ABLe Change) framework to inform the design, implementation and appraisal of systems change efforts. The framework was applied to a community change project in Michigan, US, that was seeking to transform the status quo, e.g. a fragmented service delivery system in the context of ongoing resource constraints was described [12].

Figure 3.1 shows the ABLe Change framework that puts forward that successful implementation of systems change requires a concurrent focus on both the content of the work, referred to as 'above the line' and the

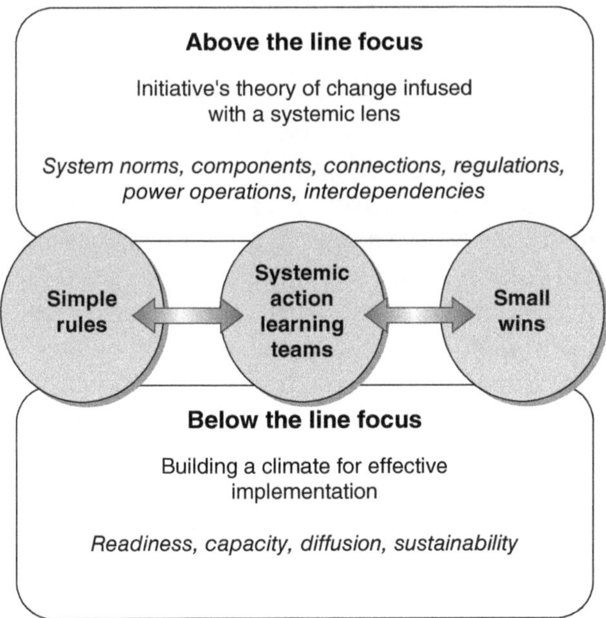

Figure 3.1 ABLe change framework [12].

Source: Reproduced with permission of Foster-Fishman and Watson [12]/ John Wiley & Sons.

processes needed, referred to as 'below the line'. A set of 'rules' that are unique to each system change effort are developed to ensure that both above and below the line content are considered.

It is evident that across the available literature, descriptions vary, and systems approaches remain poorly described. However, the definitions and concepts put forward thus far [4, 7, 9–12, 17] have undoubtedly facilitated progress towards functional reports that focus on the application of systems methods in practice. Meadows and Foster-Fishman's work is highly cited and remains greatly valued in the emerging field of implementation of systems approaches in public health and obesity, which will be discussed below.

Simple to Complex Problems

Embedding a systems way of thinking offers a deeper understanding of the drivers of complex issues such as obesity and supports a requirement to implement sustainable change through alternative, dynamic, streams of activity [4].

The 2007 Foresight Programme catalysed a paradigm shift in obesity thinking and research, putting forward that population levels of obesity are the result of over a hundred different influences and over three hundred interconnections. The 'Obesity Systems Map' – a complex web of interdependent parts – visualised obesity as a systems problem, as opposed to a simple problem with linear cause and effect. The variables were grouped across seven themes: food production, societal influences, food consumption, individual psychology, biology, individual activity and activity environment [4] (Figure 3.2).

The Foresight report fostered an improved understanding and consideration of contextual factors and dynamics such as capacity, complexity, connectivity, and social norms by conveying obesity as a challenge of a 'complex adaptive system' characterised by 'feedback loops' between at least two variables (e.g., a affects b which in turn affects a) [18]. Making clear that there is no one single cause and therefore no single solution to addressing obesity at a population level. Harry Rutter, a Professor in Global Public Health, has eminently stated 'that the single most important intervention to reduce childhood obesity is to realise that there is no single most important intervention' [19] and thus a more sophisticated approach is required.

The benefits of systems thinking include that it can assist everyone, from people living with obesity to policymakers, researchers and practitioners to have a 'bigger picture' view and explore other upstream factors, as key to tackling obesity. Lifestyle behaviour change interventions that attribute cause-effect have been the dominant response to rising obesity rates in recent decades. Where such interventions enable access to person-centred healthcare and treatment that focusses on improving

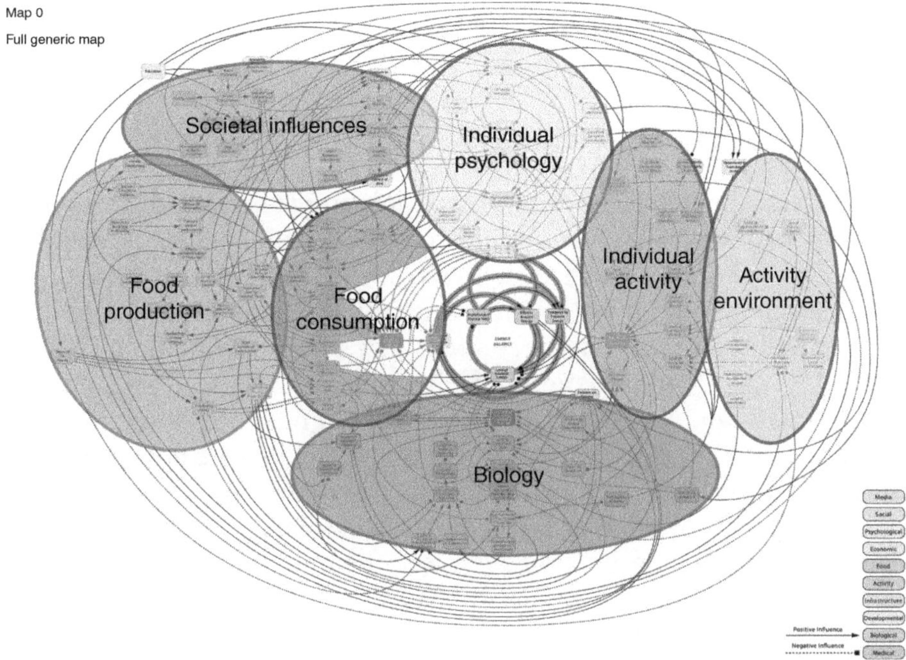

Figure 3.2 Foresight obesity systems map with thematic clusters.
Source: Adapted from [4].

overall health for people living with obesity, they remain an important 'activity' within a wider system. Indeed, systems thinking can support the design of effective individualised interventions by conceptualising them within the wider system and by considering the contribution that intervention makes to the whole obesity system in their evaluation design [4].

It is of note that the terms 'systems approach' and 'whole systems approach' are used interchangeably within the obesity literature, including a number of reports that outline key features and pragmatic examples of systems approaches to obesity within public health that have emerged in recent years [15, 20, 21] which has helped identify some common features.

A Summary of Key Features of (Whole) Systems Approaches

Broadly speaking (whole) systems approaches tend to have the following in common:

- They bring stakeholders together from multiple sectors, organisations and communities.
- They enable stakeholders to have a shared understanding of the issue and to develop a shared vision for how they can collectively change the environments in which we live.
- They are dynamic and able to adapt in response to the everchanging world that we live in.

The Application of Systems Approaches to Obesity

Implementation of Systems Approaches

There is broad scope in the implementation of systems approaches from those at a macro level; international organisations/agencies, bodies and national governments - such as those recommended by the authors of the Global Syndemic of Obesity, Undernutrition and Climate Change [22] to those operating at meso or micro level; smaller scale community-directed, illustrating transferability in application. Here, instances of system activity at a community/local level will be the focus.

As has been described earlier, systems approaches are poorly defined and often the term is used mistakenly to describe activity that in reality is several interventions being implemented in isolation. Though evidence is now starting to emerge, there remains a gap in research papers that report on **how** systems approaches to obesity are put into practice and that the research and evidence base, linked to the functioning of systems approaches in addressing complex public health issues, has not been able to keep up with the pace of implementation in the last 5–10 years [23].

In a systematic review by Bagnall et al. that included analysis of 65 process related papers exploring obesity ($n = 33$), and other complex public health issues ($n = 32$), the defining features of successful systems approaches were characterised as having full engagement with relevant stakeholders (including community), adequate funding and time to build relationships, trust and capacity, and local evaluation. Narrative synthesis of the data highlighted a lack of available evidence in how to practically operationalise a whole systems approach to obesity [24].

Building on the work of Bagnall, a review, published by Seafood in 2021, sought to better understand how systems approaches can be operationalised. Here, evidence specific to Whole Systems Approach (WSA) to childhood obesity was synthesised, and authors identified the following facilitators to implement a WSA: the need for strong leadership; allocating sufficient time to building relationships; community involvement and capacity building; ensuring consistency in language of WSA across sectors; and allocating adequate time, resource and financial support [25].

This 2021 review featured in a rapid synthesis of evidence to set out the strategic context for obesity prevention in Northern Ireland presented evidence from five existing reviews related to effectiveness of WSA in obesity prevention. Helpfully this review also offered five detailed case studies where a WSA had been applied to address obesity prevention, internationally; Shape It Up Somerville, US; Romp and Chomp and Be-Active Eat Well, Australia; Amsterdam Healthy Weight Approach and Go-Golborne, England [26].

A snapshot view of the implementation of three of the above international case studies and one additional example from the UK will follow. These real-world examples of practice-based implementation efforts that are contributing to and informing the evidence-base will be particularly useful to those who are interested in addressing population levels of obesity.

Examples from North America

COMPACT (Childhood Obesity Modeling for Prevention and Community Transformation) Study

The integration of systems science and implementation science comes together in a paper that describe the use of multiple complex systems methods to better understand a whole-of-community obesity prevention intervention called 'Shape Up Somerville' (SUS) in Massachusetts, US, which was initiated in 2002 and demonstrated sustained lower BMI z-score in intervention communities compared to control. Here, the evolution of a qualitative systems map representing community change dynamics applied retrospectively to SUS is described, and how that then informed the COMPACT study that utilised a range of complex systems tools including qualitative systems mapping, theory building and quantitative agent-based modelling and social network analysis provide a roadmap for future application [27].

Example from Australia

WHOSTOPS (Whole of Systems Trial of Prevention Strategies for Childhood Obesity)

This is a cluster-randomised trial of a systems approach to coordinating community action for childhood obesity prevention involving 10 communities in the Great South Coast region of Victoria, Australia. The aim of the trial, which started in 2015, was to test the effectiveness over a five-year period of community owned, supported and led strategies designed to address the complex and dynamic causes of childhood obesity by reporting on obesity prevalence of children aged 7–8 years, 9–10 years and 11–12 years. It involved a pilot Sustainable Eating Activity Change initiative with five communities randomised in the initial two-year period, with the remaining five joining after the second year. An external comparison group also enabled assessment of the diffusion of the intervention to control communities [28].

A paper reporting on the initial two years of the whole of community work outlines the application of systems wide approaches in the development, implementation and evaluation design. The researchers apply the earlier described framework and guiding questions by

Foster-Fishman to describe the activities and understand the systems characteristics [11]. The process of 'establishing system boundaries' and *'understanding fundamental system parts as potential root causes'* were described in the paper, and the findings were suggestive of the fact that the design and implementation of WHOSTOP in the first two years facilitated a reorientation towards a community empowered and led practice that were innovative and inspired by community-based system dynamics. It is of note that the data for the paper was based on the lived experience of community leaders of the initiatives [29].

In a process evaluation, Jenkins et al. conducted semi-structured interviews with steering group and community members and found that strong and equitable relationships between steering organisations and topic experts were key, and community and future sustainability were promoted through Asset Based Community Development.

Examples from Europe: The Amsterdam Healthy Weight Programme (AHWP) and the LIKE Programme

In Europe, Amsterdam has been leading the way in addressing childhood overweight and obesity through the promising AHWP which was conceived in 2012 and initiated in 2013 and which stems from the earlier Dutch JOGG [30] and French EPODE [31] work. The programme has a long-term vision for all children to be healthy weight in a healthy environment by 2033 and is a local area-led programme to improve children's physical activity, diet and sleep through action in the family household, local neighbourhood, school and wider city. It adopts a WSA, where the drivers of obesity are viewed as a complex adaptive system, and aims to develop interventions, apply a 'health in all policies' approach and educate professionals and target groups within the communities that are most vulnerable to child obesity, and related complex health and well-being issues [32].

The United Nations International Children's Emergency Fund (UNICEF) has stated that AHWP is trail blazing in four key areas:

1. Applying a child rights lens to equitably reach all children
2. Investing in innovative city-level programming
3. Enhancing partnership models for allocation of resources
4. Supporting professionals [33].

The LIKE programme for 10- to 14-year-old adolescents is part of the wider Amsterdam programme and uses a systems dynamics and participatory action research approach where quick (quick testing, adapting and possibly catalysing further action) and disruptive co-created

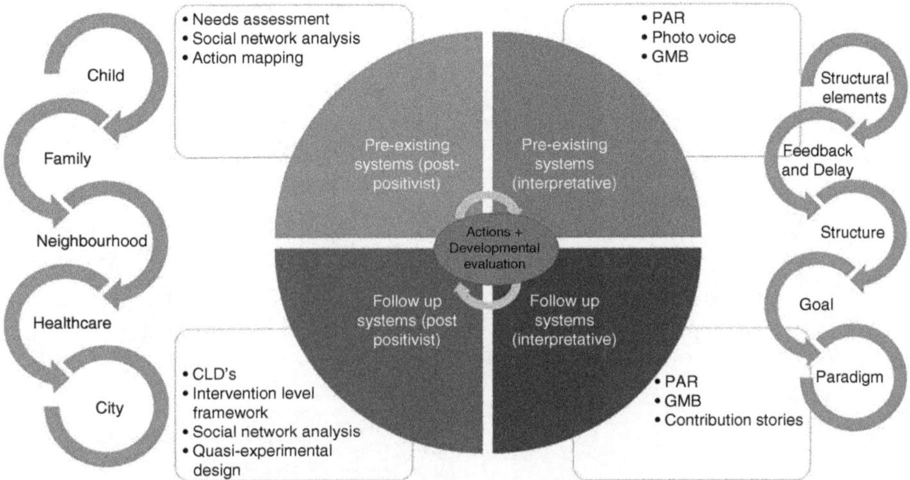

Figure 3.3 Overview of the different components of the LIKE programme and how they relate to each other. CLD, causal loop diagram; GMB, group model building; PAR, participatory action research.

Source: Wilma Waterlander [34]/MDPI/CC-BY-4.0.

actions (aiming at paradigm change or the goals of the system) that focus on function are happening at different levels of the system shown in Figure 3.3.

The LIKE programme is supported by a developmental evaluation in which an evaluation framework was developed that depicts the different components of the LIKE programme and how they relate to each other. This includes a summary of evaluation questions, related systems principles and boundaries, and specific methods to answer each question. The evaluation aims to support the development and implementation of the actions and produce generalisable knowledge, both in terms of outcome and process [34].

Crucially, the wider AHWP theory had been formally documented through development of a logic framework [35]. An example of impact evaluation [36] will be highlighted below.

Examples from the UK

The development of PHE's guide [37] proved to be a useful and practical toolkit for assisting community and stakeholder involvement in operationalising a WSA to obesity, guided by a six-phased cyclical model, shown in Figure 3.4.

The methodology (phase 1–6) facilitates a better understanding of the complex, interdependent and dynamic system that causes obesity, delivery through of a series of workshops and making use of a range of tools and resources such as causal mapping, action mapping and network analysis. Stakeholders are able to prioritise areas to intervene within the

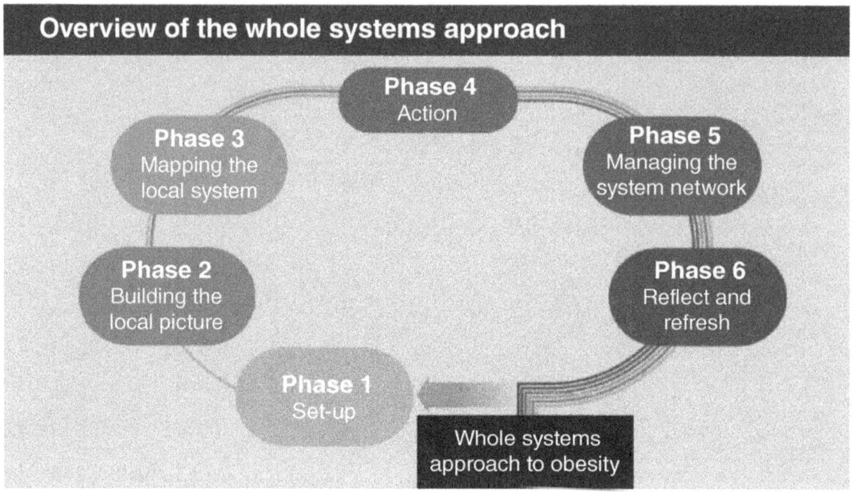

Figure 3.4 Public health England's six-phase whole systems approach.
Source: Adapted from Ref. [37].

system through collaboration and alignment of work plans. In addition, there is scope for interventions and actions to be matched against the wider determinants of health through an action mapping activity. A recently published paper has demonstrated the steps required to do this and provided examples of the visual representation that is created to highlight that many more causes of obesity are linked to wider conditions such as income equality or living and working conditions such as housing, yet very few actions (or interventions) are focussed here [38].

Crucially the publication of this guide increased access to systems techniques to public health practitioners and offered one way to implement systems approaches at a local level and enable Local Authorities to create their own local WSA. Application of this methodology was tested in seven local authorities in England between 2015 and 2017 and 5 key actions for further development in embedding a WSA were themed as follows:

- knowledge and skills related to systems thinking
- knowledge exchange and skill share
- systems leadership, communication and evaluation [39].

The Scottish Government also identified 8 local authorities areas in Scotland to implement a WSA to diet and healthy weight in 2019 [40]. A description of the process of implementation of Public Health England's six-phase methodology [37] in the midst of the Covid-19 pandemic has been described in a report [41] with case studies [42]. Nine key recommendations to advance roll-out across the country were put forward. A developmental evaluation of the early stages of a WSA in Dundee, Scotland, has been carried out and will be described below.

The current upsurge in systems approaches to address obesity that are taking place within real-world practice necessitate suitable evaluation and assessment of impact. Resource, capacity and expertise for systems evaluations are important considerations that should be embedded into any systems approach from the start.

The Evaluation of Systems Approaches to Obesity

To date, the evaluation of systems approaches to obesity has most commonly been a description and appraisal of the process of implementation as many of the above examples demonstrate. This has been extremely important in assisting practitioners and researchers with practical insights into how to operationalise approaches and to enable learning and improvement for future implementation.

The evaluation of systems approaches is very important, not least because it will help decisions about implementation and upscale. The research evidence is fast moving and emerging while only a few studies have evaluated the impact or effectiveness of systems approaches to obesity by measuring programme outcomes. A number of evaluation frameworks that have been developed will now be described.

Examples from Australia

The earlier example of the emerging work in community settings in Australia offers some rare insights into evaluation planning [31]. WHOSTOPS was significant because it was a longer trial of its type than any that had previously been undertaken and, in a rare example, the publication of implementation related data has been followed by the evaluation of four-year outcomes. The approach was found to have initially reduced overweight/obesity in the intervention group, although this increased in the following years. At four years, WHOSTOPS helped intervention children keep their takeaway food intake low and sustain Health Related Quality of Life compared with control children [43].

Examples from Europe

The Evaluation of Programmes in Complex Adaptive Systems (ENCOM-PASS) Framework was devised by researchers [36] as a means to support the evaluation of the LIKE programme for adolescents. An overview of the LIKE programme is shown in Figure 3.5. The traditional, linear processes of programme design, implementation and evaluation that puts forward pre-specified outcomes is not appropriate in systems dynamics

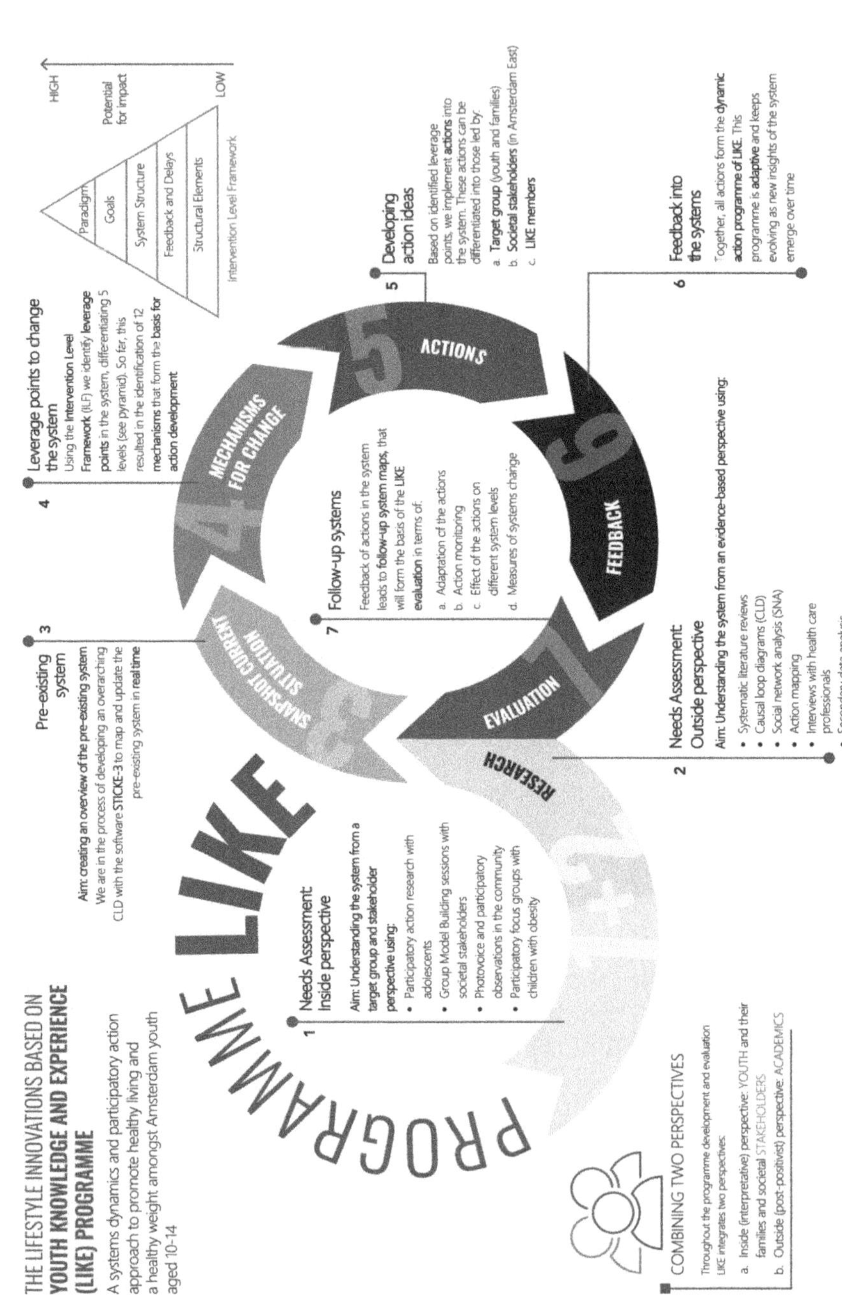

Figure 3.5 Overview of the LIKE programme.

Source: Wilma Waterlander [36]/Springer Nature/CC BY 4.0.

which must explore the wider intended or unintended impacts and their interaction with the wider context where they are taking place.

Researchers developed a five-stage iterative ENCOMPASS framework which includes the following steps: (1) adopting a system dynamics perspective on the overall evaluation design; (2) defining the system boundaries; (3) understanding the pre-existing system to inform system changes; (4) monitoring dynamic programme output at different system levels; and (5) measuring programme outcome and impact in terms of system changes with a focus on contribution and not attribution. This is shown in Figure 3.6.

Authors conclude that the value of ENCOMPASS lies in the integration of key characteristics from existing systems evaluation studies as well as in its practical application in a systems dynamic evaluation, from understanding the system, to developing actions to change the system, to measuring system changes. There is an acknowledgement that it will not be static but rather will evolve and change and that ENCOMPASS itself should be evaluated. The evaluation should appraise whether the theory described in each stage is applicable in practice; what types of results each stage generates; and how various stakeholders perceive the usefulness and legitimacy of the results.

Examples from the UK

Developmental evaluations offer a more flexible approach compared to traditional evaluations, responding to the need to support real-time learning in complex and emergent situations, where there are multiple stakeholders and high levels of uncertainty and are thus suited to systems evaluations. A key feature is that the evaluator is embedded in the initiative as a member of the team [44].

An embedded researcher helped facilitate activity in a developmental evaluation of the early stages of the implementation of a WSA (following the PHE guide) in Dundee, Scotland, and key findings of this work offers useful insights that are transferrable to other systems approaches [45]. In this example the evaluation was framed around the question: does the approach taken in Dundee support key stakeholders to recognise what they can do in relation to actions at different levels within the system? Informed by an initial evaluability assessment process and logic modelling, the research design used mixed methods including semi-structured interviews, training peer researchers to interview their wider networks, an online survey and action learning sets with key stakeholders to agree recommendations for future development and scaling of the WSA. Key findings highlighted that the WSA brought people together across different organisations and developed joint responsibilities around the priority themes, assisted stakeholders to define their roles and explore how their own activities are related to those of others. The WSA process facilitated a shared understanding of the problem and the underlying drivers

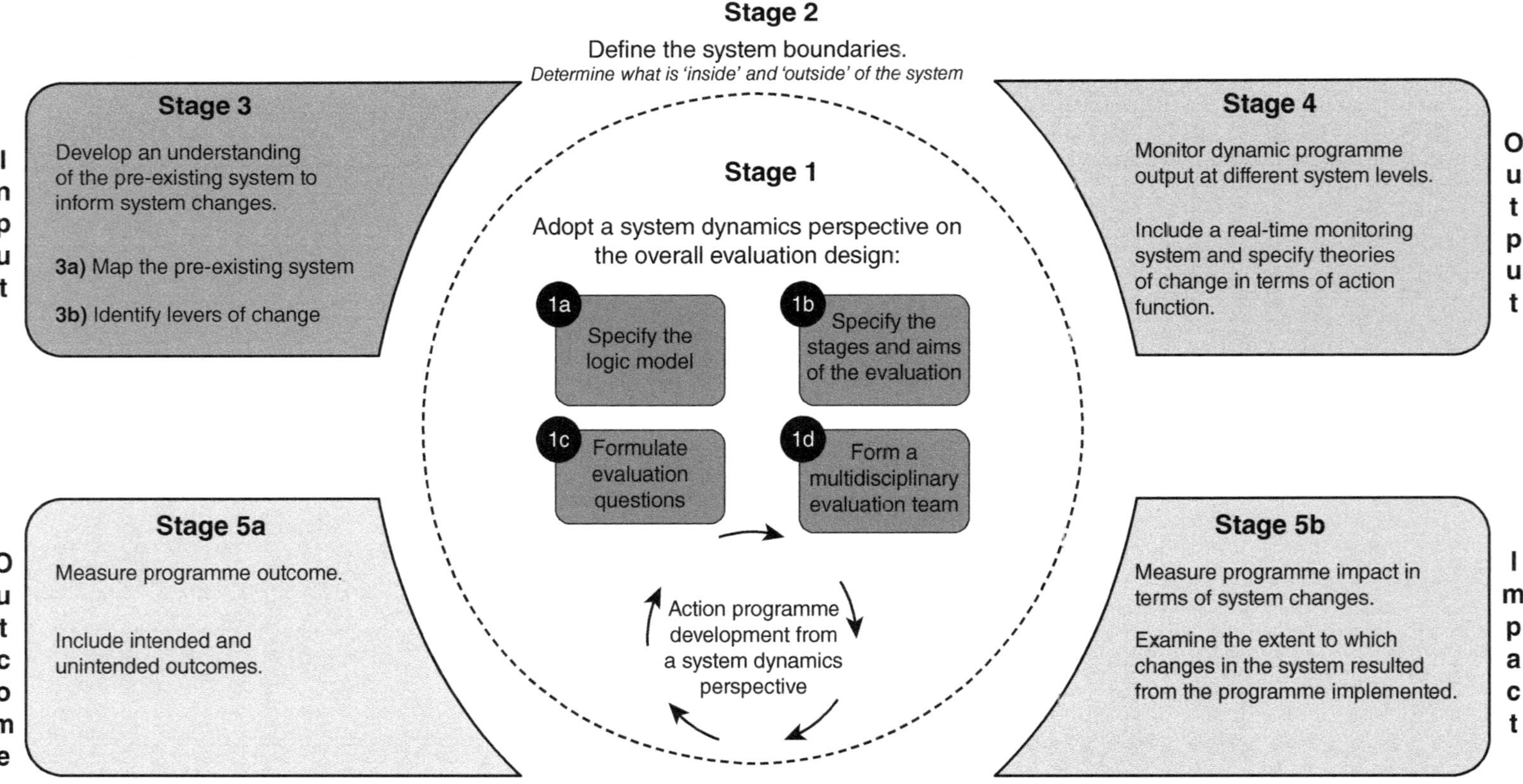

Figure 3.6 Overview of the various iterative stages in the ENCOMPASS framework.

Source: Wilma Waterlander [36]/Springer Nature/CC BY 4.0.

of childhood obesity with stakeholders. Barriers to overcome included ongoing silo-working, missed opportunities for joined-up working, few stakeholders feeling they had the influence and power to affect change and limited sustained funding. There was action planning around the concept of 'stickability': pledging as senior leaders and supporting others for ongoing leadership to embed the approach across the region through community engagement, effective messaging, aligned strategies and agendas, and evidence-based resource allocation.

In another evaluation example, the experiences and reflections of five embedded researchers, who supported four distinct WSA's to physical activity, were considered and key recommendations for researchers and commissioners who work with embedded researchers were put forward. The paper highlighted the importance of managing expectations of all stakeholders, ensuring the embedded researcher becomes integrated into the team, for example through regular meetings and debriefs. Key recommendations for the embedded researchers were curious about the local context, impartial, define boundaries and illuminate the different perspectives of stakeholders. For the commissioners, recommendations centred around having flexibility in their contracts (being open and adaptable to changes in the methods, outputs etc.) and awareness of the time required for 'academic bureaucracy' that can limit timely progress [46].

Further research and evaluation into the perceived effectiveness of systems approaches that have been implemented to address obesity in practice is needed. Non-traditional methods that better reflect the real-world setting and interaction with the local context in which interventions are delivered are required because traditional methods such as surveys, interviews or focus groups (that measure change related to pre-specified outcomes) may not account for wider impacts that may be unintended.

Ripple Effects Mapping (REM) is an example of a method that has been successfully adopted in situations where it is valuable to understand the contribution of a programme or project to the wider impacts over time [47] and can help better understand the mechanism of change that is behind the intervention effort. REM has recently been used in WSAs to public health, with authors encouraging others to make use of the approach [48]. A useful, free-to-access online training package is now available for introduction-to-ripple-effects-mapping.

Opportunities, Challenges and Future Direction of Systems Approaches to Obesity

Importantly, systems approaches can help focus collective effort around population-level actions and public health activity that address the society-wide upstream root causes, which will have greater impact on population levels of obesity at multiple levels within the system. This may include, for example, structural changes that address the food and built environment, social inequality and socio-economic disadvantage [48] or upstream interventions such as legislative or fiscal measures at an international or national level - for example the UK-wide soft drinks industry levy of 2018 resulted in reformulation of sugar sweetened beverages [49].

With the focus of this chapter being on local government and/or community-level systems activity, it is useful to highlight just one of the actions contributing to a transformational systems approach to addressing childhood obesity lead by London's Childhood Obesity Task Force [50] where restrictions on the marketing and advertising of high fat, sugar, salt foods across the transport for London network have been shown to have some positive impact [51, 52].

Similarly practice-based work carried out in Bristol, UK, to develop a local advertising and sponsorship policy [53] outlines what could be possible in terms of local action as part of a systems approach to reduce population exposure to unhealthy commodity advertising. Council-owned advertising spaces prohibited the advertising of unhealthy food and drink (HFSS), alcohol, gambling and payday loans. The National Institute for Health and Care Research (NIHR) supported ongoing evaluation of the work [54] including two paper from a team of researchers and practitioners. One paper explored the associations between measured exposure to outdoor advertising, self-reported exposure and self-reported consumption [55]; and the other explored the rationale, barriers and facilitators to implement the policy and described the perceived advertising environment prior to implementation [56].

There remains ongoing uncertainties in the evidence base related to systems approaches to address obesity [26]. A recent report looked into the issues that were limiting the use of systems approaches to improve health and address health-related inequalities such as obesity. The report identified three factors that should be considered in order to progress research in this area: a **synthesis of existing evidence** on systems-based approaches and generating new evidence to add value; **develop a global community of practice** for systems approaches in public health, to connect researchers and other key stakeholders, including policymakers and public health practitioner; **facilitate change** – funding and community – and capacity building activities [57].

Conclusion

In conclusion, this chapter has put forward that systems thinking helps account for the complexity of the causes and realities of obesity and facilitating a shared understanding of the issue. It is clear that multiple definitions and descriptions of systems approaches exist, and there are key themes of commonality. The increase in the application of systems thinking and systems approaches to address population levels of obesity over the last 10 years includes a number of highly promising international examples that were described in the earlier text. Whilst some of these systems approaches describe and evaluate the process of implementation, very few offer longer term outcome evaluation, and therefore there is a need for research and evaluation effort to focus on the impact and effectiveness of systems approaches to obesity. This can be facilitated by directing funding towards systems approaches to public health and bringing together researchers, practitioners and other stakeholders.

WHAT DOES THIS MEAN FOR PRACTICE?

Obesity is a complex and multifactorial disease with root causes that may be: biological; genetic; food and/or built environment related and linked to wider, social and commercial determinants.

- Over three decades, attempts to address obesity have focussed on individual-level, lifestyle behaviour change interventions, requiring a high degree of personal agency and government strategies to address population levels of obesity have failed.
- Systems thinking helps redress the balance by accounting for complexity and facilitating a shared understanding of the causes and realities of obesity.
- There has been an increase in the application of systems thinking and systems approaches to address population levels of obesity in the last 10 years.
- Multiple definitions and descriptions of systems approaches exist, and there are key themes of commonality.
- A number of international examples of systems approaches to obesity are now cited in the literature, some of which describe and evaluate the process of implementation.
- There is a need for research and evaluation effort to focus on the impact and effectiveness of systems approaches to obesity.

Acknowledgements

With thanks to Dr James Nobles for reviewing and sense checking earlier versions of this chapter.

References

1 Stewart, L. (2021). Personal communication: practitioner.

2 Swinburn, B. and Wood, A. (2013). Progress on obesity prevention over 20 years in Australia and New Zealand. *Obes. Rev.* 14 (S2): 60–68.

3 Theis, D.R.Z. and White, M. (2021). Is obesity policy in England fit for purpose? Analysis of government strategies and policies, 1992–2020. *Milbank Q.* 99 (1): 126–170.

4 Butland, B., Jebb, S., Kopelman, P. et al. (2007). *Tackling Obesities: Future Choices – Project Report*. London: Government Office for Science.

5 Nobles, J.D., Radley, D., and Mytton, O.T. (2021). The action scales model: a conceptual tool to identify key points for action within complex adaptive systems. *Perspect. Publ. Health* 142: `https://doi.org/10.1177/17579139211100674`.

6 Castellani, B. and Hafferty, F. (2009). Mapping complexity. *Underst. Complex Syst.* 2009.

7 Meadows, D.H. (2009). Thinking. In: *Systems* (ed. Development TIIfEa). London: Earthscan 235 p.

8 Attwood, M., Pedler, M., and Pritchard, S. (2003). *Leading Change: A Guide to Whole Systems Working*. Policy Press `https://doi.org/10.1332/policypress/9781861344496.001.000+1`.

9 Meadows DH. Leverage points: places to intervention in a system. Sustain. Inst. 1999 1–21. `https://donellameadows.org/wp-content/userfiles/Leverage_Points.pdf` (accessed 22 March 2024).

10 Meadows, D.H. (2008). *Thinking in Systems: A Primer*. Chelsea Green Publishing.

11 Foster-Fishman, P.G., Nowell, B., and Yang, H. (2007). Putting the system back into systems change: a framework for understanding and changing organizational and community systems. *Am. J. Commun. Psychol.* 39 (3–4): 197–215.

12 Foster-Fishman, P.G. and Watson, E.R. (2012). The ABLe change framework: a conceptual and methodological tool for promoting systems change. *Am. J. Community Psychol.* 49 (3): 503–516.

13 World Health Organization (2022). Systems thinking for noncommunicable disease prevention policy: guidance to bring systems approaches into practice, 1–78. `https://iris.who.int/bitstream/handle/10665/357174/WHO-EURO-2022-4195-43954-61946-eng.pdf?sequence=1` (accessed 22 March 24).

14 World Health Organization (2022). Systems Thinking for Noncommunicable Disease Prevention Policy 2022. Report No.: Technical Report: Factsheet.

15 Baugh Littlejohns, L. and Wilson, A. (2019). Strengthening complex systems for chronic disease prevention: a systematic review. *BMC Publ. Health* 19 (1): 729.

16 Academy of Medical Science CAoHS (2021). Systems-based approaches in public health: where next? 1–28. `https://acmedsci.ac.uk/file-download/73812388` (accessed 22 March 2024).

17 The Government Office for Science. Foresight Tackling Obesities: Future Choices - Project Report. Science Gof; 2007.

18 Finegood, D.T., Merth, T.D.N., and Rutter, H. (2010). Implications of the Foresight Obesity System Map for Solutions to Childhood Obesity. *Obesity* 18 (S1): S13–S16.

19 Rutter, H. (2012). The single most important intervention to tackle obesity. *Int. J. Publ. Health* 57: 657–658.

20 National Institute of Health and Care Excellence (2010). *Identifying the Key Elements and Interactions of a Whole System Approach to Obesity Prevention.* National Institute of Health and Care Excellence (NICE).

21 Garside, R., Pearson, M., Hunt, H. et al. (2010). *Identifying the Key Elements and Interactions of a Whole System Approach to Obesity Prevention.* Peninsula Technology Assessment Group (PenTAG): Exeter.

22 Swinburn, B.A., Kraak, V.I., Allender, S. et al. (2019). The global syndemic of obesity, undernutrition, and climate change: the lancet Commission report. *Lancet* 393 (10173): 791–846.

23 Nobles, J., Fox, C., Inman-Ward, A. et al. (2022). Navigating the river(s) of systems change: a multi-methods, qualitative evaluation exploring the implementation of a systems approach to physical activity in Gloucestershire, England. *BMJ Open.* 12 (8): e063638.

24 Bagnall, A.-M., Radley, D., Jones, R. et al. (2019). Whole systems approaches to obesity and other complex public health challenges: a systematic review. *BMC Public Health* 19 (1): 8.

25 Safefood (2021). Whole systems approach to childhood obesity: a review of the evidence, 1–49. https://www.safefood.net/getattachment/0627fcc9-48aa-4ab9-ac8c-d23a01aff3f9/Whole-systems-approach-to-obesity_Accessible.pdf?lang=en-IE (accessed 22 March 24).

26 Breslin, G.W.W., McGowan, L., Mack, J.B. et al. (2022). *A Whole Systems Approach to Obesity Prevention: A Rapid Synthesis of Evidence to Inform the Northern Ireland Obesity Prevention Strategy Project Board.* Dublin: Institute of Public Health.

27 Hennessy, E., Economos, C.D., Hammond, R.A. et al. (2020). Integrating complex systems methods to advance obesity prevention intervention research. *Health Educ. Behav.* 47 (2): 213–223.

28 Allender, S., Millar, L., Hovmand, P. et al. (2016). Whole of systems trial of prevention strategies for childhood obesity: who stops childhood obesity. *Int. J. Environ. Res. Public Health* 13 (11): 1143.

29 Allender, S., Brown, A.D., Bolton, K.A. et al. (2019). Translating systems thinking into practice for community action on childhood obesity. *Obes Rev.* 20 (Suppl 2): 179–184.

30 Van Koperen, T.M., Jebb, S.A., Summerbell, C.D. et al. (2013). Characterizing the EPODE logic model: unravelling the past and informing the future. *Obes. Rev.* 14: 162–170.

31 Borys, J.M., Le Bodo, Y., Jebb, S.A. et al. (2012). EPODE approach for childhood obesity prevention: methods, progress and international development. *Obes. Rev.* 13 (4): 299–315.

32 den Hertog, K. and Busch, V. (2020). The Amsterdam Healthy Weight Approach: a whole systems approach for tackling child obesity in cities. *Eur. J. Publ. Health* 30 (Supplement_5): ckaa165.516.

33 UNICEF (2020). *City of Amsterdam, EAT, The Amsterdam Healthy Weight Approach: Investing in Healthy Urban Childhoods: A Case Study on Healthy Diets for Children.* © United Nations Children's Fund (UNICEF). UNICEF.

34 Waterlander, W.E., Luna Pinzon, A., Verhoeff, A. et al. (2020). A system dynamics and participatory action research approach to promote healthy living and a healthy weight among 10–14-year-old adolescents in Amsterdam: the LIKE programme. *Int. J. Environ. Res. Public Health* 17 (14): 4928.

35 Sawyer, A., den Hertog, K., Verhoeff, A.P. et al. (2021). Developing the logic framework underpinning a whole-systems approach to childhood overweight and obesity prevention: Amsterdam Healthy Weight Approach. *Obes. Sci. Pract.* 7 (5): 591–605.

36 Luna Pinzon, A., Stronks, K., Dijkstra, C. et al. (2022). The ENCOM-PASS framework: a practical guide for the evaluation of public health programmes in complex adaptive systems. *Int. J. Behav. Nutr. Phys. Act.* 19 (1): 33.

37 Public Health England (2019). Whole Systems Approach to Obesity: A Guide to Support Local Approaches to Promoting a Healthy Weight. Report No.: PHE Publications Gateway Number GW-534.

38 Nobles, J., Christensen, A., Butler, M. et al. (2019). Understanding how local authorities in England address obesity: a wider determinants of health perspective. *Health Policy (Amsterdam, Netherlands)* 123 (10): 998–1003.

39 Public Health England (2019). *Whole systems approach to obesity programme. Learning from co-producing and testing the guide and resources.* London: Public Health England.

40 Obesity Action Scotland (2023). Whole systems approach early adopter areas 2023. `https://www.obesityactionscotland.org/wsa/introduction-to-whole-system-approaches-wsa/wsa-in-scotland/` (accessed 22 March 24).

41 Public Health Scotland (2022). *Whole Systems Approach (WSA) to Diet and Healthy Weight: Early Adopters Programme Process Evaluation.* Public Health Scotland.

42 Public Health Scotland (2022). *Whole Systems Approach(WSA) to Diet and Healthy Weight: Early Adopters Programme Process Evaluation: Case Studies.* Public Health Scotland.

43 Allender, S., Orellana, L., Crooks, N. et al. (2021). Four-year behavioral, health-related quality of life, and BMI outcomes from a cluster randomized whole of systems trial of prevention strategies for childhood obesity. *Obesity (Silver Spring)* 29 (6): 1022–1035.

44 Dozois, E.L.M. and Blanchet-Cohen, N. (2010). *A Practitioner's Guide to Developmental Evaluation.* The J.W. McConnell Family Foundation and the International Institute for Child Rights and Development.

45 van der Graaf P MH, Subramanian M, O'Malley C, Lake A, Gillespie J, Cook W, Passey A & Chng NR. An Evaluation of 'Healthy Weight Tayside', a whole system approach to child healthy weight in Dundee City 2022 [NIHR131566]. `https://fundingawards.nihr.ac.uk/award/NIHR134419` (accessed 22 March 2024).

46 Potts, A.J., Nobles, J., Shearn, K. et al. (2022). Embedded researchers as part of a whole systems approach to physical activity: reflections and recommendations. *Systems* 10 (3): 69.

47 Chazdon, S., Emery, M.E., Hansen, D. et al. (2017). *A Field Guide to Ripple Effects Mapping*. Minneapolis, MN: University of Minnesota Libraries Publishing.

48 Nobles, J., Wheeler, J., Dunleavy-Harris, K. et al. (2022). Ripple effects mapping: capturing the wider impacts of systems change efforts in public health. *BMC Med. Res. Methodol.* 22 (1): 72.

49 Rogers, N.T.C.S., Forde, H., Jones, C.P. et al. (2023). Associations between trajectories of obesity prevalence in English primary school children and the UK soft drinks industry levy: an interrupted time series analysis of surveillance data. *PLoS Med.* 20 (1): e1004160.

50 Taskforce LsCO (2019). *Every Child a Healthy Weight: Ten Ambitions for London*. © Greater London Authority.

51 Thomas, C., Breeze, P., Cummins, S. et al. (2022). The health, cost and equity impacts of restrictions on the advertisement of high fat, salt and sugar products across the transport for London network: a health economic modelling study. *Int. J. Behav. Nutr. Phys. Act.* 19 (1): 93.

52 Policy TA (2019). *Approval Guidance Food and Non-Alcoholic Drink Advertising*. Transport for London `https://content.tfl.gov.uk/policy-guidance-food-and-drink-advertising.pdf` (accessed 22 March 2024).

53 Bristol City Council (2021). Advertising and Sponsorship Policy 2021. `https://democracy.bristol.gov.uk/documents/s58004/Appendix%20Ai%20-%20Advertising%20and%20Sponsorship%20Policy.pdf` (accessed 22 March 2024).

54 de Vocht, F.N.J., Scott, L., Jago, R. et al. (2022). *Reducing Population Exposure to Unhealthy Commodity Advertising: Evaluation of the Bristol Advertising and Sponsorship Policy (Pre-intervention Data Collection)*. National Institute for Health and Care Research (NIHR) Open Research `https://openresearch.nihr.ac.uk/documents/3-9/pdf`.

55 Scott, L.J., Toumpakari, Z., Nobles, J. et al. (2023). Assessing exposure to outdoor advertisement for products high in fat, salt and sugar (HFSS); is self-reported exposure a useful exposure metric? *BMC Publ. Health* 23 (1): 668.

56 Scott, L.J., Nobles, J., Sillero-Rejon, C. et al. (2023). Advertisement of unhealthy commodities in Bristol and South Gloucestershire and rationale for a new advertisement policy. *BMC Publ. Health* 23 (1): 1078.

57 Jebb, S.F.D., Roux, A.D., Rutter, H. et al. (2021). *Systems-Based Approaches in Public Health: Where Next?* The Academy of Medical Sciences & Canadian Acasemy of Health Sciences.

4 Raising the Topic of Child Weight

Laura Stewart

'I can't bear to raise it, and I don't want to make things worse'. [1]

Introduction

Raising the topic of a CYP's weight is without doubt a sensitive conversation [2–4]. It is such an important issue for a CYP healthy weight strategy and pathway that it is given a whole chapter within this book. It is an area that is viewed as being difficult to undertake, and many professionals are uncomfortable with raising the topic [4–6]. However, a successful strategy of managing CYP healthy weight requires appropriate discussions to take place between families and those who refer into the childhood weight management services – called gatekeepers throughout this chapter and book. Therefore, this chapter is particularly pertinent for those professionals as part of the wider CYP healthy weight team who are gatekeepers into the management pathway and for those who manage the pathway and need to consider their role in training their potential gatekeepers.

Parental Recognition

There is an abundance of evidence that demonstrates that many parents do not recognise their own child's weight status, even when their child's weight sits in the overweight and obesity categories [7–10]. This is one of the reasons that raising the topic of a CYP's weight with families can be sensitive [5]. As discussed in previous chapters, maternal weight is one of the biggest predictors of childhood obesity and therefore the mother's own weight may be seen by the health care professional (HCP) as a barrier

Child and Adolescent Obesity: A Practical Approach to Clinical Weight Management,
First Edition. Edited by Laura Stewart.

to raising the topic of the child's weight. Highlighting the importance that no implication of blame or judgement should be conveyed by the HCP [11]. For some parents, their own experiences from childhood can lead to them naturally being protective in trying to avoid stigmatisation for their child [12]. We should also not forget that media headline can often appear to be directly blaming parents for their child's weight adding to the societal sensitivity of the topic [5]. While as more of the population move into the overweight or obesity categories, this can normalise overweight in childhood making raising the topic harder [13].

Parents can be well aware of the social and psychological implications of a child's weight and in particular stigmatisation and bullying [13]. Indeed Mikhailovich et al. suggests that this may be more important to parents than the physical comorbidities associated with childhood and adult obesity [11].

> *'It's a stigma, and stigma shouldn't be placed on children'*
> *(Participant, Hardy et al. [2]).*

The HCP needs to distinguish between the problem and the patient. It is important for the HCP to explore their own attitudes and core value around this topic during clinical supervision, including improving their knowledge around the complex societal determinants of childhood and adult obesity.

In a qualitative study discussing parents views on a paediatric weight management programme, Stewart et al. developed a typology of parents prior to entering a child healthy weight service [14]. They classified parents into three typologies of *'seekers', 'avoiders' or 'deniers'*.

- The **'avoiders'** were those who recognised that their child was in the unhealthy weight category but for a variety of reasons, mainly to do with not upsetting their child, they had chosen not to discuss the issue and not to actively seek help.
- The **'deniers'** were parents who had not recognised that their child's weight was outside of the healthy weight category.
- The **'seekers'** were parents who were actively seeking advice and help to manage their child's weight [14].

While this typology does not help to pinpoint which parents will effectively engage with a service, it does help to demonstrate the need for professionals raising the issue to be well trained and understand the emotional complexities of the situation. Indeed, the HCP may be the first person to discuss the subject and the parents might have never before perceived their child's weight as outside of the healthy weight or as an 'issue' requiring them to take action. Interestingly, when seeking help, it is mothers who are usually the driving force [14, 15].

Stigma and Weight Bias

Before going any further in this chapter, this is the ideal point to return to considering stigma and weight bias, as this thread is one of the fundamental reasons that discussing weight can be a difficult to raise. Although there is limited research on weight stigma in children, Haqq et al. stated that one of the main situations were children come across weight stigma is in the healthcare setting [16]. This is indeed a shocking comment to read and tells us that everyone involved in supporting children and adults with weight management need to be more proactive in ensuring a supportive environment.

The WHO Europe gives us the two following useful definitions. First, for weight bias:

> *'Weight bias is defined as negative attitudes towards, and beliefs about, others because of their weight. These negative attitudes are manifested by stereotypes and/or prejudice towards people with overweight or obesity'* [17].

And for weight stigma:

> *'Obesity stigma involves actions against people with obesity that can cause exclusion and marginalisation and lead to inequalities'* [17].

It is good to keep these definitions in mind, not only while reading the rest of this chapter and book, but also in the context of everyday life and the working environment. The WHO Europe paper quotes statistics of 63% of school aged children with obesity experiencing a higher chance of being bullied, 54% of adults with obesity having reported stigma from co-workers, with 69% of adults with obesity having faced stigmatisation from health care professionals [17].

Haqq et al. gives us a very helpful list of the types of behaviours by others which constitute weight stigma and bias. These include:

- *'Weight bias teasing*
- *Bullying*
- *Criticising*
- *Harassing*
- *Victimisation*
- *Differential treatment leading to social exclusion, marginalisation, social inequality and adverse health outcomes'* [16].

The literature tells us that weight bias and stigmatisation tends to come from a person's overly simplistic view of the causes of weight gain and obesity, which in turn can reinforce a discourse of blame and shame [16–18]. We live in an obesogenic environment with complex factors resulting in weight gain [19], these can often be overlooked or indeed not fully understood resulting in the belief that self-control and self-responsibility for choices are the root causes. These types of attitudes have been 'called out' over the past few years with the negative impact they cause highlighted [20].

In CYP this is often seen as bullying and teasing which can in turn lead to low self-esteem and quality of life [15, 21]. Often those experiencing weight stigma internalise their feelings leading to self-directed shaming and self-devaluation [16, 17]. It is reported there can often be a belief, by those demonstrating weight stigma and bias, that the shaming should encourage weight management behaviours [21]. However, people who have experienced weight stigma frequently report participating in what appears to be counterintuitive behaviours such as eating more to cope reporting a spectrum of overeating behaviours, reduced eating self-efficacy and avoidance of physical activity [21–23]. With negative effects on both physical and mental health including depression [23].

In young people, Pont noted that the bullying and teasing associated with weight can lead to low self-esteem, poor body image, social isolation, including school avoidance with diminished academic achievements [21]. It would appear that weight stigma and bias could potentially stem from anyone including family, friends, peers, educators, healthcare providers and for adults work colleagues, with the media often a source of reinforcing the stereotypical prejudices [16, 17, 21]. This is a long list of people who could display weight stigma and bias, and it is not hard to understand how hearing this consistently can have such a negative effect.

Use of Language

There is an overwhelming breadth of evidence that using the words *'overweight'* or *'obese'* to describe a CYP's weight with families and CYP can lead to stigma, shame and guilt [12, 24, 25]. This knowledge along with a huge push by patients groups, such as the European Coalition of People Living with Obesity (ECPO – www.eurobesity.org), to coin and promote the term 'people first' language [17, 20, 26]. With people first language the person is related to as just that – a person and not by their disease/illness. Therefore, someone with diabetes is a person with diabetes or a person living with diabetes and not a diabetic. Similarly, a person with overweight or obesity is a person living with overweight or obesity and not obese or overweight. There is also a move to avoid the depersonalisation photos of only showing parts of people with obesity to showing the whole person and not showing stereotypical poses such as eating a large burger and chips [17]. There is a suite of photos of people of all ages, genders and ethnicity free to use at www.worldobesity.org/resources/image-bank, which aims to tackle weight bias in photos used worldwide in all arenas.

Although the preferred term for adults is a person living with obesity, there is a subtle but important difference when talking about CYP. The American Academy of Pediatrics (AAP) expert report of 2007, their policy statement on stigma (2017) and the Clinical Practice Guidelines (2023) recommend the more neutral terms of *weight, unhealthy excess weight* and *BMI* when discussing with the topic parents or CYP. It is worth noting that they still suggested using the more clinical terms of *overweight* and *obesity* within clinical documentation [20, 21, 24].

Parents interviewed by Hardy et al. said that they did not want the HCPs to use words such as *fat, chubby, chunky or obese* [2, 11]. In Mikhailovich's work, *weight, BMI* and *overweight* were preferred by parents. Whereas Brown and Flint found that parents preferred the terms *weight, unhealthy weight* and *BMI* for describing their child's weight. Other suggestions would include *healthy weight, fitter, leaner* and *lighter* [12, 20, 21, 25]. Terms that seem to be consistently disliked and can evoke strong negative feelings in parents include *fat, extra-large* and *extremely obese* [20, 24, 25]. Whichever of these preferred terms you choose to use with parents, CYP and families, it is important to ensure that the whole team and even gatekeepers to the service try to use the same terms to ensure consistency.

Discussing Difficult to Hear Topics

There is an abundance of evidence to support that Health and Social Care Professionals (H&SCPs) can find it uncomfortable to convey what is often termed 'bad' or 'difficult' news [4, 13, 27]. Professionals should expect a wide range of responses including both positive and negative reactions from parents [11]. Although this chapter is about discussing the topic of child weight, there is much that can be learnt from HCPs raising difficult news in other contexts. Brouwer et al. and Levetown give excellent reviews of paediatric HCPs communicating with parents and families across a number of difficult situation such as informing the parents of their child's diagnosis of life threatening cancer [27, 28]. Much, if not all, that they discuss is pertinent to our discussion on child healthy weight.

Communicating in a client or family centred manner is essential to establishing rapport and building a trustful relationship between the HCP, parent and child [28]. This has been described as building a partnership which helps to facilitate the parent and child feeling comfortable to express their own concerns and suggestions, allowing them the time and space to tell their own story [28]. With empathy and a non-judgemental approach being effective in promoting communication [13, 28], all combine to facilitate joint, shared decision-making and client centredness. Levetown noted that the attitudes from the HCP that are predictive factors of effective communication include their:

- Perception of interest
- Caring attitude
- Warmth
- Responsiveness [28].

The impact of a communication style should not be underestimated and, although discussed further in Chapter 5, is briefly outlined here. Part of this is the development and use of active listening skills. This is essential for all HCP and especially for those working with CYP living with obesity and their families. This is a skill that requires practicing in a face to face or online workshop type learning environment. It is good to consider and practice using the useful acronym OARS, especially when discussing a sensitive issue such as weight and previous weight management attempts. It is essential for language to be appropriate and sensitive, and by using OARS we will structure the conversation is a sensitive, person-centred way.

> **OARS** = **O**pen questions
> **A**ffirmations
> **R**eflections
> **S**ummaries

Open Questions
- Establish and build a trusting and respectful relationship.
- Explore, clarify and gain an understanding of the CYP/parent's world.
- Learn about the CYP/parent's past experience, feelings, thoughts, beliefs, and behaviours.
- Gather information – allow the CYP/parent to do most of the talking.
- Help the CYP/parent make an informed decision.

Affirmation – acknowledging past achievements, the person's strengths and efforts.

- Builds rapport, demonstrates empathy.
- Affirm exploration into the CYP/parent's world.

- Affirm the CYP/parent's past decisions, abilities and healthy behaviours.
- Build self-efficacy – an ability to believe they can be responsible for their own decisions and their lives.

Reflection – reflective listening: repeating, rephrasing and paraphrasing. Reflecting both the words used and the feelings conveyed by the CYP/parent. Various types of reflections:

- Simple reflections
- Amplified reflections
- Double-sided reflections
- Reflection of emotion

Helpful ways to begin reflections include

- "You . . ."
- "It sounds like you . . ."
- "So you . . ."
- "It seems to you that . . ."
- "You are wondering if . . ."
- Demonstrates that you are listening and trying to understand the situation.
- Offers the CYP/parent an opportunity to 'hear' their own words, feelings and behaviours reflected back.
- Reflect the CYP/parent's thoughts, feelings and behaviours.
- Reflect the CYP/parent's general experiences and the 'in the moment' experience.

Summarising
- Keeps you and the CYP/parent on the same page through the session.
- Summarises the session will help close the session with an agreed plan of action.

Raising the Topic of a Child's Weight

Some countries work within a weight screening programme, with the CYP having their weight and height measured at school. BMI is calculated and an indication of the meaning of the BMI is sent to the parents. As an example visit National Child Measurement Programme – NHS Digital. In this programme, the CYP has their measurements taken twice during the primary years of education, at ages 4–5 years and then at 10–11 years.

Grimmett et al. found that of those parents surveyed, 65% welcomed the feedback and wished that their child's weight was monitored on a regular basis. They also found there to be no adverse effects for the CYP from having the measurements taken at school [29]. Although this English system and one seen in Arkansas, US (<u>Arkansas Center for Health Improvement – ACHI</u>), appear to be acceptable, they are not widely replicated.

Discussion on the topic of a child's weight often sits within complex family situations, which may include issues such as safe guarding, emotional or behavioural problems, competing family demands or lack of parental acceptance [13]. It cannot be over-emphasised that communicating in an empathetic and non-judgemental manner is exceedingly important in building the trusting, collaborative, relationship between the parents and health care system and supporting the subsequent decision-making [2, 11].

In many countries the role of discussing weight with parents and families sits firmly with school/paediatric nursing. A 2019 study by Sjunnestrand et al. found that paediatric nurses felt that a major barrier to them addressing childhood obesity with parents was actually organisational factors, including not having ongoing training for this role and no clear referral pathway [4, 6]. Many of the HCPs appeared reluctant to raise the topic for fear of offending the parent [4, 13] and of receiving positive or negative reactions [2, 13]. Many parents found their child's weight a sensitive topic associated with stigma and negative feelings [13]. It can also be seen as more 'difficult' topic to raise if the parents themselves are perceived to have overweight or obesity [2, 4] and when parents have different perception of their child's weight [2]. Often HCPs prefer to not damage their ongoing relationship with the parent and family and thus may rather avoid raising the topic of the child's weight [5]. While there is also quite a few studies which highlight that the HCPs' own weight status can influence how they perceive raising the topic of weight as a challenge [11, 13]. All underlining the importance of supporting those raising the topic to reduce the missed opportunities to raise the topic and support the family [4].

Some HCPs have been found to lack understanding around the complexities of the issue, lack confidence, feel intimated and importantly insufficiently trained [13]. It is therefore important to ensure that gatekeepers to services have the necessary knowledge around the local pathway and have the required organisational support to feel comfortable discussing the topic, including awareness of the societal stigma around weight [6, 13]. It has been recommended that it is important for this training to be included in ongoing Continuing Professional Development (CPD) [2]:

> *'There are many principles of good communication, including positivity, being helpful and supportive, being collaborative and understanding'* [30].

What has been found helpful by parents when the topic was raised includes:

- Using open-ended questions
- Using a BMI chart
- Interplay with parents, a good relationship
- A recognised and joined-up pathway
- Showing concern, confidence and care
- Having time for questions
- Giving written information
- Valuing the child
- Conveying an attitude of no guilt, blame or judgement
- Showing concern rather than detachment
- Allowing plenty of time for questions
- Respecting the parent [4, 11].

In considering the Brouwer, HCP–parent–CYP relationship [2, 13, 27], in the context of CYP weight management, the parents *intimate knowledge* of their own child should complement the work of the HCP. Many parents want a clear weight management care plan with a holistic approach [2], with the role of the HCP to offer evidence-based information within a non-judgemental support context [2, 13].

Parents wish the discussion to take place with them first, so they can decide what is best for their child [5]. Reid found that parents considered it less challenging to have discussions around levels of physical activity rather than what types of foods their child ate. Interestingly, she also found that discussing portion sizes of food was acceptable to parents [5]. Cultural contexts, including language and parental beliefs and values, are very important to take into consideration when discussing this topic [12, 13, 27, 28].

PHE has produced a very relevant and helpful document called 'Let's Talk about Weight: A step-by-step guide to conversations about weight management with CYP and families for health care professionals' [3]. This is a valuable document for anyone whose work will include discussing CYP's weight and for those training others. It relates to discussions concerning children aged 4–12 years, but many aspects will be relevant to both younger and older age groups. It discusses the need to use an objective measurement and not simply visually identifying weight status, see below, while also noting the importance of using professional judgement of the appropriate timing and place for raising the subject of CYP's weight [3].

PHE have recommended a process of using 'three As' for a structured conversation process, the three As being – ASK, ADVISE and ASSIST. Table 4.1 gives a few example of language that could be used in this

Table 4.1 Ask, advise, assist.

ASK	'How worried are you about Daisy's weight?'	'Would it be okay if I checked Daisy's weight and height today?'	'Tell me about Daisy's activity levels through the week'
ADVISE	'Let me show you where Daisy sits on this chart. This shows that she is sitting outside the healthy weight range.'	'I'll give you this leaflet about the services available in your area to support you, Daisy and the family.'	'We know from working with other families and young people that they find our weight management programme to be really helpful'
ASSIST	'Our weight management programme helps you and Daisy make small lifestyle changes. How do you feel about that?'	'How do you feel about what we have discussed today?'	'This might not be the right time for you and Daisy and that is fine. Just come back and let us know when you feel ready.'

Source: Adapted from Hardy et al. [2].

process. Remember that open ended questions are important for opening up conversations and making the interaction person centred, [5] for example *'How do you feel about Daisy's weight?'* Whereas, closed interviewing techniques can be perceived as showing a lack of interest in the person [11, 28]. Empathetic, non-judgemental approaches encourage a positive and favourable response while a more authoritarian approach can elicit anger [13].

Parents can be unsure what to do and how to move forward once the topic has been raised [2]. Therefore, it is important that those HCPs delivering this news have the appropriate communication skills, knowledge of local pathways and understanding of health literacy. Information should be given in writing and/or signposting to good, reliable online information [5].

It is vital to use concrete information with parents when discussing their children's weight status. BMI plotted correctly on a physical chart or in an online tool is the best method to use [12, 24, 31]. When choosing which BMI tool will be used across a service and by gatekeepers, it is important to ensure that the background population normative data is the correct data for your population. For example, an online tool from the US is not appropriate to be used with a UK population as US background population normative data will have been used and not UK data. Here is an example of an online tool for plotting BMI using UK data: `Calculate your body mass index (BMI) – NHS – NHS (www.nhs.uk) (www.nhs.uk)`. See Chapter 8 for more in-depth discussion on the use and interpretation of BMI and BMI tools in CYP weight management.

A systematic review exploring the parental role in discussing weight and related issues with their children was carried out by Grey et al.. They found that this could have positive influences for the CYP if there was already a foundation of solid parent–child communications which was characterised by warmth and openness. Many parents felt less confident about being the person to initially raise the conversation and that this was influenced by how knowledgeable the parent felt on the topic of weight, weight management and the appropriate language to use [32]. It can help the CYP with the talk with their parents if there is no blame or negative language used regarding the CYP's body weight and shape. Exploring the topic and discussing this with a look towards becoming healthier can feel more supportive to the young person. During development of the UK WATCH-IT programme, qualitative interviews were undertaken with the CYP who had gone through the programme. The CYP noted that they felt that their parents had delayed discussing weight and they had been waiting for the parent to raise the topic [15, 33].

Health Literacy

This leads to finishing off this chapter by stating the importance of being aware of health literacy. Health literacy can be described as *'having the appropriate skills, knowledge, understanding and confidence to access, understand, evaluate, use and navigate health and social care information and services'* [34].

Health literacy as discussed by Nutbeam includes communication and interactive literacy in its widest sense. It includes consideration of cognitive and social skills [35]. These skills can influence and determine a person's ability and motivation to engage with health services. It is therefore important to be aware of the cultural, social and health literacy background of the individuals and groups the service is engaging with around child healthier weight.

Weight management services should consider that individual conversations on a child's weight should not sit in isolation from local public health messages and service gatekeepers' knowledge of these messages. Some public health departments may have an expert in health literacy and they will be an excellent person to make contact with for help around written materials and approaches to discussing the topic of child weight.

WHAT DOES THIS MEAN FOR PRACTICE?

It is important to ensure that there is high quality and readily available training for all health professionals and gatekeepers working in the area of child healthy weight. The evidence certainly supports that this should include ongoing training on the overall subject and in raising the topic. This training should include plotting and interpreting BMI and the use of any BMI tools which are being considered locally. Any online BMI tools need to be relevant to your countries' BMI population, using the correct population norms for the background calculation.

It is vital to have an agreed, clear and local clinical pathway, ensuring that training involves information on this local clinical pathway and that there is available supporting literature. Literature on services designed for the population and potential client families should be checked for appropriate reading age and be in the relevant cultural languages of your population. Take into account the importance of avoiding stigmatising language, terms and photographs in any programme or service literature.

Within a service team, it would be good practice to use individual supervision for exploring individual attitudes, values and beliefs towards people living with obesity. While for the team as a whole, it is important to explore all their processes, programme, programme materials and training to ensure promoting non-stigmatising language and terms is seen as the service norm.

References

1 Gillespie, J., Midmore, C., Hoeflich, J. et al. (2015). Parents as the start of the solution: a social marketing approach to understanding triggers and barriers to entering a childhood weight management service. *J. Hum. Nutr. Diet.* 28: 83–92. https://doi.org/10.1111/jhn.12237.

2 Hardy, K., Hooker, L., Ridgway, L. et al. (2019). Australian parents' experiences when discussing their child's overweight and obesity with the Maternal and Child Health nurse: a qualitative study. *J. Clin. Nurs.* 28: 3610–3617. https://doi.org/10.1111/jocn.14956.

3 Public Health England (2017). Let's talk about weight: a step-by-step guide to conversations about weight management with children and families for health and care professionals. https://assets.publishing.service.gov.uk/government/uploads/system/uploads/attachment_data/file/649095/child_weight_management_lets_talk_about_weight.pdf (accessed 29 March 2024).

4 Sjunnestrand, M., Nordin, K., Eli, K. et al. (2019). Planting a seed-child health care nurses' perceptions of speaking to parents about overweight and obesity: A qualitative study within the STOP project. *BMC Publ. Health* 19. https://doi.org/10.1186/s12889-019-7852-4.

5 Reid, M. (2009). Debrief of a study to identify and explore parental, young people's and health professionals' attitudes, awareness and knowledge of child healthy weight.

6 Turner, G.L., Owen, S., and Watson, P.M. (2016). Addressing childhood obesity at school entry: qualitative experiences of school health professionals. *J. Child Heal. Care* 20: 304–313. https://doi.org/10.1177/1367493515587061.

7 Jeffery, A.N., Voss, L.D., Metcalf, B.S. et al. (2005). Parents' awareness of overweight in themselves and their children: cross sectional study within a cohort (EarlyBird21). *Br. Med. J.* 330: 23–24. https://doi.org/10.1136/bmj.38315.451539.F7.

8 Etelson, D., Brand, D.A., Patrick, P.A. et al. (2003). Childhood obesity; do parents recognize this health risk? *Obes. Res.* 11: 1362–1368.

9 Lundahl, A., Kidwell, K.M., and Nelson, T.D. (2014). Parental underestimates of child weight: a meta-analysis. *Pediatrics* 133: e689 LP–e703 LP. https://doi.org/10.1542/peds.2013-2690.

10 Regber, S., Novak, M., Eiben, G. et al. (2013). Parental perceptions of and concerns about child's body weight in eight European countries – the IDEFICS study. *Pediatr. Obes.* 8: 118–129. https://doi.org/10.1111/j.2047-6310.2012.00093.x.

11 Mikhailovich, K. and Morrison, P. (2007). Discussing childhood overweight and obesity with parents: a health communication dilemma. *J. Child Heal. Care* 11: 311–322. https://doi.org/10.1177/1367493507082757.

12 Chadwick, P. and Croker, H. (2015). Talking about weight with families. In: *Early Years Nutrition and Healthy Weight* (ed. L. Stewart and J. Thompson), 59–70. Wiley.

13 Bradbury, D., Chisholm, A., Watson, P.M. et al. (2018). Barriers and facilitators to health care professionals discussing child weight with parents: a meta-synthesis of qualitative studies. *Br. J. Health Psychol.* 23: 701–722. https://doi.org/10.1111/bjhp.12312.

14 Stewart, L., Chapple, J., Hughes, A.R. et al. (2008). Parents' journey through treatment for their child's obesity: a qualitative study. *Arch. Dis. Child.* 93: 35–39. https://doi.org/10.1136/adc.2007.125146.

15 Murtagh, J., Dixey, R., and Rudolf, M. (2006). A qualitative investigation into the levers and barriers to weight loss in children: opinions of obese children. *Arch. Dis. Child.* 91: 920–923. https://doi.org/10.1136/adc.2005.085712.

16 Haqq, A.M., Kebbe, M., Tan, Q. et al. (2021). Complexity and stigma of pediatric obesity. *Child. Obes.* 17: 229–240. https://doi.org/10.1089/chi.2021.0003.

17 World Health Organization (2017). Weight bias and obesity stigma: considerations for the WHO European Region. WHO-EURO-2017-5369-45134-64401-eng.pdf (accessed 30 March 2024).

18 Chadwick, P., Sacher, P., and Swain, C. (2014). Talking to families about overweight children. *Br. J. Sch. Nurs.* 3: 271–276. https://doi.org/10.12968/bjsn.2008.3.6.31696.

19 Butland, B., Jebb, S., Kopelman, P. et al. (2007). Tackling obesities: future choices – project report. *Foresight* 162: https://doi.org/10.1002/hep.20263.

20 Hampl, S.E., Hassink, S.G., Skinner, A.C. et al. (2023). Clinical practice guideline for the evaluation and treatment of children and adolescents with obesity. *Pediatrics* 151: e2022060640. https://doi.org/10.1542/peds.2022-060640.

21 Pont, S., Puhl, R., Cook, S. et al. (2017). Stigma experienced by children and adolescents with obesity. *Pediatrics* 140: e20173034. https://doi.org/10.1542/peds.2017-3034.

22 Lessard, L.M., Puhl, R.M., Himmelstein, M.S. et al. (2021). Eating and exercise-related correlates of weight stigma: a multinational investigation. *Obesity* 29: 966–970. https://doi.org/10.1002/oby.23168.

23 Flint, S.W. (2021). Time to end weight stigma in healthcare. *EClin. Med.* 34: 100810. https://doi.org/10.1016/j.eclinm.2021.100810.

24 Barlow, S.E. (2007). Expert committee recommendations regarding the prevention, assessment, and treatment of child and adolescent overweight and obesity: summary report. *Pediatrics* 120: S164–S192. https://doi.org/10.1542/peds.2007-2329c.

25 Brown, A. and Flint, S.W. (2021). Preferences and emotional response to weight-related terminology used by healthcare professionals to describe body weight in people living with overweight and obesity. *Clin. Obes.* 1–9. https://doi.org/10.1111/cob.12470.

26 Albury, C., Strain, W.D., Le, B.S. et al. (2020). The importance of language in engagement between health-care professionals and people living with obesity: a joint consensus statement. *Lancet Diabetes Endocrinol.* 8: 447–455. https://doi.org/10.1016/S2213-8587(20)30102-9.

27 Brouwer, M.A., Maeckelberghe, E.L.M., Van Der Heide, A. et al. (2021). Breaking bad news: what parents would like you to know. *Arch. Dis. Child.* 106: 276–281. https://doi.org/10.1136/archdischild-2019-318398.

28 Levetown, M. (2008). Communicating with children and families: from everyday interactions to skill in conveying distressing information. *Pediatrics* 121: https://doi.org/10.1542/peds.2008-0565.

29 Grimmett, C., Croker, H., Carnell, S. et al. (2008). Telling parents their child's weight status: psychological impact of a weight-screening program. *Pediatrics* 122: https://doi.org/10.1542/peds.2007-3526.

30 Albury, C., Le Brocq, S., Lloyd, C. et al. (2020). Language matters: obesity. Obesity-Language-Matters-_FINAL.pdf (easo.org) (accessed 30 March 2024).

31 Stewart, L. (2008). Recognizing childhood obesity: the role of the school nurse. *Br. J. Sch. Nurs.* 3: 323–326. https://doi.org/10.12968/bjsn.2008.3.7.31714.

32 Grey, E.B., Atkinson, L., Chater, A. et al. (2022). A systematic review of the evidence on the effect of parental communication about

health and health behaviours on children's health and wellbeing. *Prev. Med. (Baltim.)* 159: 107043. https://doi.org/10.1016/j.ypmed.2022.107043.

33 Dixey, R., Rudolf, M., and Murtagh, J. (2006). WATCH IT: obesity management for children: A qualitative exploration of the views of parents. *Int. J. Heal. Promot. Educ.* 44: 131–137. https://doi.org/10.1080/14635240.2006.10708085.

34 Public Health England and UCL Institute of Health Equity (2015). Improving health literacy to reduce health inequalities. 4b_Health_Literacy-Briefing.pdf (publishing.service.gov.uk) (accessed 30 March 2024).

35 Nutbeam, D. (2000). Health literacy as a public health goal: a challenge for contemporary health education and communication strategies into the 21st century. *Health Promot. Int.* 15: 259–267. https://doi.org/10.1093/heapro/15.3.259.

5 Changing Behaviours

Laura Stewart

'It was like forming a partnership and it worked'. [1]

Introduction

Changing and then maintaining lifestyle behaviour is complex, difficult and challenging for most people. That is why it is important to consider approaches and tools to help facilitate and support behaviour change [2]. The purpose of this chapter is to explore and discuss using a person and family-centred approach to facilitate behaviour change. Changing behaviour is not always easy, if it was there would not be a need for a professional to help the CYP and their family to navigate their purposed changes and help plan how to implement them. Being able to support behaviour change is a skill which can be learnt and needs to be practiced.

In childhood weight management, behavioural change techniques are deployed to help the young person and their parents to consider the necessary changes they need to make and to transverse the obesogenic environment. Healthier lifestyle behaviours are influenced by a multitude of factors including family, the environment, community, kinship groups and local policies [3]. Managing weight requires modifications to be made to an individual's energy balance utilising behavioural changes strategies [4]. There are three main areas of lifestyle that need to be explored in modifying any individual's energy balance [1]. These are looked at in more depth in other chapters and are quickly noted here as:

- Reducing the total energy intake from food and drinks (Chapter 7)
- Increasing physical activity (Chapter 6)

Child and Adolescent Obesity: A Practical Approach to Clinical Weight Management,
First Edition. Edited by Laura Stewart.
© 2024 John Wiley & Sons Ltd. Published 2024 by John Wiley & Sons Ltd.

- Decreasing time spent on screen time (sedentary behaviours) (Chapter 6).

The necessary lifestyle changes and the use of behaviour change techniques to facilitate change should sit within a defined weight management programme. This programme may be group based, 1:1 consultations or indeed a mixture of group and 1:1 sessions delivered within a variety of settings by a range of potential HCPs [5]. The behavioural changes techniques and strategies discussed in this chapter can be utilised within both group and 1:1 programmes. It is worth noting that 1:1 consultations give room and scope to help both explore and support more complex situations [5, 6], whereas groups help to give a sense of peer support. Some programmes may use a combination of group and 1:1 sessions. All programmes are deemed to be more successful if they are delivered by a multi-disciplinary team [7].

In this chapter, we are not discussing any particular programme, but the potential behavioural modification aspects that should be utilised within any programme. This chapter has been written with the expectations that these behavioural change techniques would be delivered within a defined programme that is tailored to individual needs; that is delivered with consistent fidelity by well-trained HCPs [8, 9]. Practicing all these techniques in a training, safe environment is the ideal way to learn to use these tools effectively and proficiently.

We discuss in other chapters throughout this book the types of training and interpersonal skills required of HCP working in the field of CYP weight management. It is worth considering here the necessary qualities and attributes of HCPs in this field:

- Non-judgemental
- Effective communicator
- Empathic
- Ability to establish rapport
- Friendly engaging demeanour
- Ability to work with people
- Charisma
- Viewing a non-pathological lens on obesity
- Enthusiasm for the field of childhood obesity management [5].

A Person-Centred Approach

Using a person-centred behavioural approach to weight management has become the approach of choice in recent years among professionals and underpins the use of the behavioural change techniques discussed in this chapter [2, 10]. It takes as a starting point the experiences and opinions of the person wishing to make the changes. It is also child friendly and child focused [1]. The HCP should not be seen as the expert telling a person what to do but enabling them to explore their reasons for change and supporting them in planning and implementing their plan for change. The supportive, non-judgemental and positive attitude of the HCP has been noted as important for the continued engagement of young people and their families [1, 11].

In childhood weight management, to whom the behavioural change is directed at depends on the age of the CYP. There are no firm rules; however, clinical practice would suggest the following ages for directing the conversation:

- Under eight to ten years the behaviour change is aimed at the parents
- From eight to ten years until early teenage years, it is aimed predominately at the young person with considerable parental support
- From thirteen/fourteen years onwards, it is aimed at the young person with the parent in a supporting role. The parent may even be out of the room for a part of the conversation, but always brought back in to confirm any potential changes agreed with the young person [12].

In a person-centred, family-based approach, it is important to encourage the support of the family and establishment of a social support network [4, 13], working towards flexible and gradual changes in lifestyle [4]. That means that the CYP are not the only person within the family network who is making any changes to their lifestyle. Role modelling of proposed changes is seen as essential.

Listening Skills

An essential element to successfully using behaviour change techniques is to be an effective listener and to use active listening skills [14]. These skills have been discussed in Chapter 4 and are expanded here using the mnemonic – OARS.

- **O**pen questions
- **A**ffirmations
- **R**eflections
- **S**ummarising [15].

Open Questions

An open question is one that cannot be answered as a yes/no. *'Was it a good day at school today?'* could be answered as yes or no. *'Tell me about your day at school'* leaves the recipients open to tell the answer in any way that seems important to them. They can give as long or as short an answer as suits them, leaving the person asking the questions room to further follow-up questions and to clarify what they have heard.

Using open questions is an important way of sharing information, and ensuring the consultation is a two-way conversation. People (of any age) generally feel more involved in the process and it helps to support establishing a shared agenda and a person-centred approach [11, 15]. In weight management, these are important in keeping the young person, parents and family engaged and also ensuring that the process is a positive experience.

Instead of asking *'So, you are here today about your weight?'*

Say *'Tell me your reasons for coming today'*.

The second question is more open and allows the young person or parent to give and explore their reasons for attending. While closed questions give the participant a limited way to answer, there are certain occasions within a conversation with children and young people where a well-placed closed question is suitable and indeed may be desirable.

Affirmations

Affirmations give the person answering positive feedback for their actions; they show that the listener is actually listening to what matters to the speaker. Affirmations are a means of acknowledging achievements, strengths, effort and abilities [15]. We all appreciate praise and well-placed affirmations during a consultation help to support and build rapport between the young person/parents and the HCP. Affirmations also help to build self-efficacy by supporting an inner self-belief.

'It's really good that you came today'.

'You have managed to increase your activity to walking 20 minutes on 4 days a week, that's such an improvement since last time we talked'.

'Thanks for bringing your lifestyle diary today, it's really good that you and your mum took the time to fill this out'.

Reflections

Using reflective listening involves repeating back to the young person or parent their words or short phrases sometime as rephrasing or paraphrasing. Reflecting can include both the words used and the feelings conveyed by the clients.

'You're feeling happy today'

'That seems to have annoyed you'.

The use of reflections demonstrates that you are listening and trying to understand the situation from the young person or parent's perspective. It presents the young person or parent with an opportunity to 'hear' their own words, feelings and behaviours reflected back. Well-used reflections are less likely to stir a defensive response [15].

There are various types of reflections that can be used throughout a consultation and these include:

- Simple reflections: *'meal times are difficult for you'*.
- Amplified reflections: *'it sounds like you can never see chocolate without eating it'*.
- Double-sided reflections: *'It seems like you enjoy eating chocolate but afterwards it makes to feel frustrated with yourself'*.
- Reflection of emotion: *'You sound as if you are feeling sad today'*.

Helpful ways to begin reflections include:

- *'You are feeling ...'*
- *'It sounds like you ...'*
- *'It seems to you that ...'*

Summarising

Summarising as you go throughout a session helps to keeps the HCP and the young person or parent *'on the same page'* through the session. Short summarises can be helpful to aid clarification of what the young person or parent is telling. They can also be used as a summary of the session so far and help with moving the conversation onto the next stage. Finally, summarising of the pertinent points of the whole session will help close the session with an agreed plan of action.

Building Rapport

The ability of the practitioner to build and establish a rapport with the young person, their parents and family is considered to be an essential aspect of making the intervention a person-centred and positive experience [6]. Building a rapport involves developing a therapeutic relationship built on being non-judgemental and displaying empathy [6, 14]. Showing an interest in the whole person and not being solely focused on weight can further aid the HCP in building rapport. In qualitative feedback from child weight management programmes, parents often talk about feeling they are part of a partnership when they have formed a rapport with the HCP [16].

Initially forming a rapport can involve simple interactions:

- Introducing yourself
- Asking who everyone in the room is and their relationship with the CYP
- Making small talk about the weather or something the CYP is wearing such as colourful trainers
- Being open and honest.

Establishing a Shared Agenda

This is an important concept which supports the HCP's attempts to be being person-centred and establish rapport with their patients. Establishing a shared agenda should be one of the initial aspects of the consultation, establishing that everyone is there for the same reason – of managing the weight of the CYP [14]. It is not unheard of for parents to be more concerned about other aspects of their child's lifestyle such as sleep pattern or for them to be attending because they *'have been told to'* by another professional and are not themselves concerned about their child's current weight. Therefore, it is a good starting point to ask the parent or parents and young person to *'tell me your reason for coming here today'*.

Through information exchange and by utilising good listening skills, a shared agenda will emerge during the programme of the types of agreed behaviour changes that are required, acceptable and realistic.

Managing Expectations

An exceedingly important aspect of behaviour change and developing rapport is managing expectations. Much of this will be discussed in the first consultations, but should also continue throughout the programme. Managing expectations will include discussions and clarity on:

- Length, number and frequency of sessions
- An outline of what the particular programme entails e.g. goal setting, a person-centred approach, concurrent physical activity sessions
- An outline of behaviour changes required i.e. changes to energy being taken in, increasing physical activity levels, decreasing screen time

- Expectations of weight outcome from the programme (see Chapter 8) i.e. weight staying the same and height growth or small weight loss for some teenagers
- Or weight outcome not being a main factor and other aspects such as decrease in blood sugar levels, being able to undertake activity without being breathless

Talking through the expectations of the above helps the young person and parents to decide if this is the right programme for them and if this is the right time to engage in the programme for them. It helps to build the foundations of a partnership and of them feeling they are in control of the process and its outcomes.

Talking through the expectations of weight outcomes as early as possible is essential. If a young person and their family think that by decreasing chocolate by one bar a day will result in a weekly weight loss, then they will be disappointed when this does not occur and will most likely leave the programme. Therefore, discussing the realistic expectations of for example weight staying the same is important for them to perceive success of the programme. Weight expectations in a childhood programme are discussed in more depth in Chapter 8.

Behaviour Change Theories

There are many theories of behaviour change that underpin smoking cessation, alcohol reduction and weight management programmes [2]. It is not the intention of this chapter to explore the various theories, but to give a brief overview of the two most important behavioural change theories that most frequently underpinned childhood weight management programmes [5], and those being the transtheoretical model of change (also known as the model of change) [17] and social cognitive theory [18].

The Transtheoretical Model of Change

The transtheoretical model of health change was originally postulated by Prochaska and Di Clemente in the 1980s [17]. This model construes behavioural change not as a single event but as a fluid process with five main stages – the stages of change. These five changes, which are briefly outlined below, are often represented in a circle (see Figure 5.1) and that a person may follow the change model in any given order or direction, such as moving from action on dietary change back to precontemplation.

> *Precontemplation* – not intending to take any action, often measured within the next three to six months.

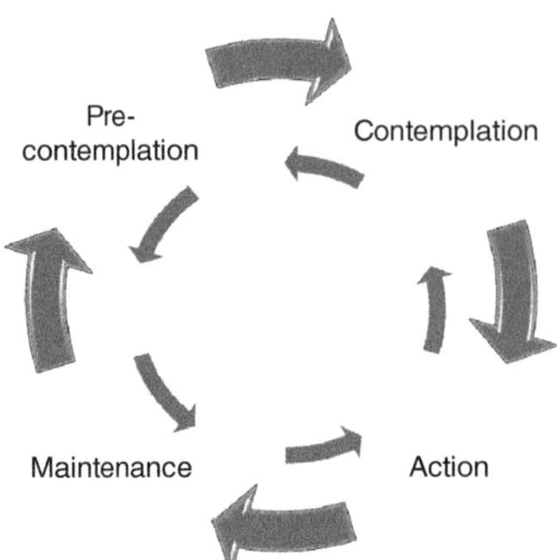

Figure 5.1 Representation of the model of change.

Source: Adapted from [19].

Contemplation – intending to change in the next three to six months.

Preparation – intending to take action in the immediate future, i.e. within the next month.

Action – specific, intended changes in lifestyle have been undertaken.

Maintenance – working to prevent relapse of behaviour.

Social Cognitive Theory

Social cognitive theory originally proposed by Bandura suggests that an individual's capability to change a specific behaviour is 'learnt' through observation, thus the importance of role modelling. There needs to be a perceived and acknowledged outcome expectation such as weight staying the same, being able to walk further. In making a decision about what to change they need to have expectations of their ability to achieve the new behaviour. Finally, the individual requires reinforcements for achieving the new behaviour such as feeling better, a new magazine or a sticker on a chart [18].

It is easy to see how the tools of problem solving, goal setting, modelling and exploring past change attempts are all used to help increase self-efficacy and positive reinforcement for change.

Behaviour Change Tools

There are a number of behaviour change strategies that are commonly used throughout childhood weight management programmes. These are derived from the above theories as well as other behaviour change theories. In the main these are

- Exploring motivation
- Goal setting

- Use of rewards
- Self-monitoring
- Behavioural incentives
- Environment/Stimulus control
- Preventing relapse [2, 4, 5, 9, 20].

Exploring Motivation

A powerful tool to use at the beginning, and at other points, in a programme is to explore motivation of the young person and their parents [15].

Importance of change can be examined by using a simple 1–10 scaling [14]. The young person and parent may give a number on a scale from 0 to 10 to describe how important it is for them to make change or get the CYP's weight under control.

> *'It would be really helpful if you could give me an idea of how important it is to you to get your weight under control/to you to get your child's weight under control. Using 0 to 10 where 0 means it is not important to you at all (and you can put 0), 5 means important but not the most important thing to you and 10 is very important to you right here and right now. And you can say any of the numbers in-between. Where would you put yourself/your child on this scale?'*

Although simple, this tool can be exceedingly useful in opening conversations around weight management and possible barriers to making lifestyle changes. Another useful tool often used at the same point as the importance scale would be to use a simplified decisional balance chart (sometimes call an ambivalence chart) [14]. This exercise helps the young person and parent to focus on the positive reasons for making lifestyle changes. It is usual to start with the good things and then finish with the not so good things.

- *'What would be the good things about getting your/Johnny's weight under control?'*
- *'What would be not so good about making some of these lifestyle changes?'*

Keep asking the questions until you are sure that all possible answers have been given [21]. Summarise both sides of the change position using the young person's or parent's own words. Always summarise back, starting with the not so good things so that you end with the list of good things.

It is helpful to take the not so good side of the decisional balance chart to view each perceived 'problem' in turn and discuss possible ways in which they could be overcome. For example, to explain to a young person who has concerns over *'never being able to eat crisps again'* that they will not have to give up all crisps and that they will be in control of their own goal setting during the programme. The good things about getting the weight under control are their internal reasons for wishing to change and are good to refer back to and even revise during the programme.

Self-Monitoring

Self-monitoring involves the young person or parent recording their current lifestyle. It has been shown to be one of the most effective behavioural change tools [22, 23]. Its usefulness lies in it being a tool that helps to increase awareness of current lifestyle and then helps to monitor their ability to keep to current lifestyle change goals [1]. Self-monitoring should never be seen as just looking at dietary intake as this makes diet seem the most important factor. Therefore a lifestyle dairy that looks at the three aspects of the energy balance (or more factors) – dietary intake, physical activity levels and time spent on screens – provides a better overall picture [4, 24]. Some people also recommend recording sleep, for older teenagers' mood may even be considered.

Depending on the age of the CYP, the parent may have to take the responsibility for any recordings. It is always nice if the young person and the parent discuss the lifestyle monitoring. There are now many useful apps and tools for recording such as dietary recording apps on phone, wearable activity recorders and even taking photographs using a mobile phone [25]. What works best for the young person and the family can be discussed and then utilised.

As this is called self-monitoring, it is important for the HCP to realise that the purpose of the monitoring is not to bring or send the recording back to them to review. Yes, it can help with conversations around goal setting if it is brought to programme sessions, but that should never be seen as the main purpose of this tool. It should also be recognised that the recording of a full lifestyle diary can become burdensome [1] and a more simplistic method should be deployed to help families at around one month into a programme.

Goal Setting

The concept of setting goals should be explained to the young person and parent at the initial session, as this helps with managing expectations for the programme and with establishing a shared agenda.

In a person-centred approach, it is essential that ideas come from the young person or parent (see age-appropriate interactions above), with interaction with the young person and parent or parent and child as appropriate. The role of the HCP is <u>not</u> to offer solutions but to facilitate problem-solving over possible goals. Time within the consultation should be allowed for the young person or parent to identify a range of possible options. Setting goals is one of the times when allowing short periods of silence can help the young person or parent contemplate possible goals. In practice, parents often help their child to explore options. When there is a struggle to come up with any options, refer back to the energy balance concept and, if available, to their lifestyle diary. In a person-centred approach, the HCP can help the young person or parent explore options for change by using the person-centred friendly technique of the 'patient in the back pocket'.

'Some families/boys and girls have found it useful to ....'

At the initial setting of goals, try not to overload with numerous goals for change. It is essential that the goals are SMART:

- **S**pecific (also think Small)
- **M**easurable
- **A**chievable
- **R**ecorded
- **T**ime-phased.

As each goal is being discussed, it is important to also review possible barriers to change such as parties, holidays, wet weather. The goals can then be refined to make them more realistic. For example, a child who has identified a goal of *'never eating chocolate again'* may change this to *'only eating sweets at the weekends'* and that during holidays this goal may have to be altered. The HCP should explore the CYP and parents' confidence in their ability to achieve their goals by asking questions like:

'How sure are you that you will be able to keep sweeties to the weekend only?'

Keep refining the goal until the young person and parent feel it is realistic and they are confident they can meet it.

'Three days a week Johnny will have up to 4 sweeties'.

'Two days a week Johnny will have at least 20 minutes of active time'.

When setting goals, the HCP needs to appreciate and accept that there will be resistance to change. The practitioner needs to 'roll with the resistance' by using reflective listening, shared decision-making and if necessary, move on from a goal that upon exploration does not seem achievable [14].

Agreeing Rewards

Not all programmes will use rewards as a behavioural change tool, but they can be helpful in reinforcing behavioural change. They could be used as a tool to help increase and maintain motivation. Rewards should also involve praise and encouragement from parents and family members. In a programme, the CYP may be rewarded for reaching 100% of every goal set. The reward is discussed and agreed between the child and parent, then as with the goals are recorded. The HCP's role here is to ensure that the reward is small, affordable and importantly not food or screen time related e.g. magazine, staying up late one night per week. The parent should agree to give their child this reward if the CYP reaches 100% of all their goals. *And* the CYP needs to be aware that they will not receive their reward unless they achieve *all* their goals.

This connection between goals and rewards can help some CYP to be more realistic in setting goals. Some programmes may use a sticker chart in which a sticker is given for meeting a target and x number of stickers are required per week to 'earn' a reward as reinforcement of change.

Reviewing Goals and Rewards

If available, a lifestyle diary can be part of the discussion with the parent or young person to ascertain whether their set goals have been met. There are a number of possible scenarios which can determine the subsequent conversation in a review session.

1. If all agree that all the goals have been met and this is reflected in the recordings, then the CYP should receive their agreed reward. The young person or parent should then be asked to explore further options for extending their goals. They could keep their present goals and can either expand these, for example a goal of eating fruit every second day could be increased to eating fruit every day, or create a completely new goal.

2. If the CYP has not met 100% of their goals, then they should be praised for those goals that they have achieved. It is essential to look at the reasons that goals have not been achieved and to problem solve how to overcome the barriers to make lifestyle changes. After this, existing goals should be refined, or completely new ones made. This discussion will take place regardless of what has happened to the CYP's weight. It should never be seen as a failure to move on from a goal that has not been met. Indeed, this is being realistic and person-centred.

Depending on how frequently weight and height are measured in the programme, the weight change will also influence the conversation. A weight increase needs to be spoken about in a non-judgemental manner, for example:

> *'We need to find what is the right change in energy balance is for you Daisy.'*

On occasion through the programme the decisional balance chart and the importance of making a change might need to be revisited to help re-explore flagging or fluctuating motivation.

Environmental/Stimulus Control

This is usually part of problem-solving goals and is a way of encouraging changes in the environment to help to either reduce a behaviour or promote a new behaviour. Examples of reducing a behaviour would be to remove and reduce the amount of crisps kept in a kitchen cupboard or avoiding buying certain foods. Promoting new behaviours may be to have a football or other activity object situated prominently near the front door to encourage its use after school or at weekends or putting out fresh fruit at a level easy to reach for the CYP.

Preventing Relapse

If we consider the transtheoretical model of change [17], then we are aware that a person's motivation and importance to make behavioural changes can vary. Therefore, an important tool to be used in any programme is helping young people and parents consider planning for *'tricky or difficult situations'*. Figure 5.2 gives some ideas of what can be called potential tricky/difficult situation for a young person or parents to keep to goals,

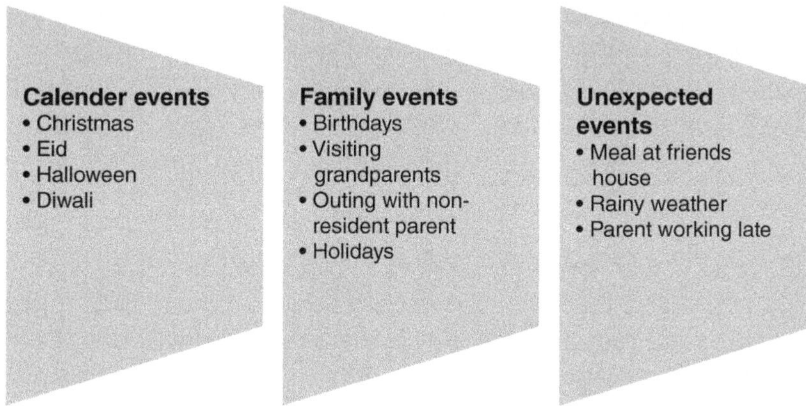

Figure 5.2 Potential tricky/difficult situations.

such as birthday parties, rainy weather and visiting relatives. This is not an exhaustive list but here for illustration of types of events which may require planning with the young person and parents.

Planning for a tricky/difficult situation can involve modifying goals in the run up to Christmas or Eid for example. Or it can involve exploring ways of mitigating the particular situation, for example having fewer high energy foods the day before or undertaking more physical activity on the day of or day after a lunch at the grandparents' house. In rainy weather where a set goal of walking cannot be met, then problem solve around what type of physical activities could reasonably be done indoors or set a goal that is weatherproofed by agreeing *'be active for at least 30 minutes 3 days per week'*. When planning for tricky/difficult situations, remember that the *'patient in the back pocket'* can be very helpful.

Patient in the back pocket is a useful technique of offering a suggestion from the point of view of the experience of others in similar situations. For example *'other boys and girls have found it helpful to reduce their number of snacks the day before going to a party. How does that sound like something you would want to do?'*

Another aspect of preventing relapse when someone's motivation may be waning would be to revisit the importance of getting weight under control and the decisional balance chart. Both these tools are helpful to revisit and help a young person or parent reassess their motivation.

WHAT DOES THIS MEAN FOR PRACTICE?

It is important that any childhood weight management programme includes the use of behavioural change tools. The programme should be delivered by a multi-disciplinary team that has been trained to use the tools effectively and appropriately for this group. HCP should utilise effective listening skills to ensure that they work in as a partnership with the CYP and their families. Developing rapport, a shared agenda and managing expectations are all elements that a well-trained, experienced practitioner will do as part of the programme they are delivering.

Facilitating person-centred, SMART goal setting is a skill that should be used throughout a weight management programme to help support the CYP and their parents to make effective behavioural changes that can be achieved and maintained.

References

1 Stewart, L., Chapple, J., Hughes, A.R. et al. (2008). The use of behavioural change techniques in the treatment of paediatric obesity: qualitative evaluation of parental perspectives on treatment. *J. Hum. Nutr. Diet.* 21: 464–473. https://doi.org/10.1111/j.1365-277X.2008.00888.x.

2 NICE (2014). Behaviour change: individual approaches. www.nice.org.uk/guidance/ph49 (accessed 01 April 2024).

3 Heerman, W.J., Jaka, M.M., Berge, J.M. et al. (2017). The dose of behavioral interventions to prevent and treat childhood obesity: a systematic review and meta-regression. *Int. J. Behav. Nutr. Phys. Act.* 14: 1–10. https://doi.org/10.1186/s12966-017-0615-7.

4 Wilfey, D.E., Hayes, J.F., Balantekin, K.N. et al. (2018). Behavioral interventions for obesity in children and adults: evidence-based, novel approaches and translation into practice. *Am. Psychol.* 73: 981–993. https://doi.org/10.1037/amp0000293.Behavioral.

5 Sahota, P., Wordley, J., and Woodward, J. (2010). Literature review-health behaviour change models and approaches for families and young people to support HEAT 3: Child Healthy Weight Programmes. http://eprints.leedsbeckett.ac.uk/817/ (accessed 29 March 2024).

6 Stewart, L., Easter, S., and BDA's Obesity Specialist Group (2021). British Dietetic Association's Obesity Specialist Group dietetic obesity management interventions in children and young people: review & clinical application. *J. Hum. Nutr. Diet.* 34: 224–232. https://doi.org/10.1111/jhn.12834.

7 NICE (2013). Managing overweight and obesity among children and young people: lifestyle weight management services PH47. guidance.nice.org.uk/ph47 (accessed 01 April 2024).

8 NHS Health Scotland (2019). Standards for the delivery of tier 2 and tier 3 weight management services for children and young people in Scotland.

9 Stewart, L., Reilly, J.J., and Hughes, A.R. (2009). Evidence-based behavioral treatment of obesity in children and adolescents. *Child. Adolesc. Psychiatr. Clin. N. Am.* 18: 189–198. https://doi.org/10.1016/J.CHC.2008.07.014.

10 Department of Health (2001). The expert patient: a new approach to chronic disease management for the 21st century. *Dis. Manag.* .

11 Pollak, K.I., Alexander, S.C., Tulsky, J.A. et al. (2011). Physician empathy and listening: associations with patient satisfaction and autonomy. *J. Am. Board. Fam. Med.* 24: 665–672. https://doi.org/10.3122/jabfm.2011.06.110025.

12 Stewart, L., Gillespie, J., and Young, T. (2017). Obesity: childhood. In: *Public Health Nutrition* (ed. J.L. Buttriss, A.A. Welch, J.M. Kearney, et al.), 205–213. Wiley Blackwell.

13 Bagherniya, M., Taghipour, A., Sharma, M. et al. (2018). Obesity intervention programs among adolescents using social cognitive theory: a systematic literature review. *Health. Educ. Res.* 33: 26–39. https://doi.org/10.1093/her/cyx079.

14 Rollnick, S., Mason, P., and Butler, C. (1999). *Health Behaviour Change: A Guide for Practitioners*. Edinburgh: Churchill Livingstone.

15 Miller, W.R. and Rollnick, S. (2012). *Motivational Interviewing: Helping People Change (Applications of Motivational Interviewing)*, 3e. New York: The Guildford Press.

16 Stewart, L., Chapple, J., Hughes, A.R. et al. (2008). Parents' journey through treatment for their child's obesity: a qualitative study. *Arch. Dis. Child.* 93: 35–39. https://doi.org/10.1136/adc.2007.125146.

17 Prochaska, J.O. and Diclemente, C.C. (1986). Toward a comprehensive model of change. In: *Treating Addictive Behaviors: Processes of Change* (ed. W.R. Miller and N. Heather), 3–27. Boston, MA: Springer US http://doi.org/10.1007/978-1-4613-2191-0_1.

18 Bandura, A. (1977). *Social Cognitive Theory*. Engelwood Cliff, NJ: Prentice Hall.

19 Prochaska, J.O. and Velicer, W.F. (1997). The transtheoretical model of health behavior change. *Am. J. Heal. Promot.* 12: 38–48. https://doi.org/10.4278/0890-1171-12.1.38.

20 Stewart, L. and Smith, C. (2020). Obesity in childhood. In: *Clinical Paediatric Dietetics* (ed. V. Shaw), 472–485. Oxford: Wileys-Blackwell. http://doi.org/10.1002/9781119467205.

21 Lask, B. (2003). Invited commentary motivating children and adolescents to improve adherence. *J. Pediatr.* 3476: 430–433.

22 Burke, L.E., Wang, J., and Sevick, M.A. (2011). Self-monitoring in weight loss: a systematic review of the literature. *J. Am. Diet. Assoc.* 111: 92–102. https://doi.org/10.1016/j.jada.2010.10.008.

23 Vallis, M., Macklin, D., and Russell-Mayhew, S. (2020). Effective psychological and behavioural interventions in obesity management. https://obesitycanada.ca/guidelines/behavioural (accessed 29 March 2024).

24 Stewart, L., Houghton, J., Hughes, A.R. et al. (2005). Dietetic management of pediatric overweight: development and description of a practical and evidence-based behavioral approach. *J. Am. Diet. Assoc.* 105: 1810–1815. https://doi.org/10.1016/j.jada.2005.08.006.

25 Burke, L.E., Conroy, M.B., Sereika, S.M. et al. (2011). The effective self-monitoring on weight loss and dietary intake: a randomized behavioral weight loss trial. *Obesity (Silver Spring)* 19: 338–344. https://doi.org/10.1038/oby.2010.208.

6 Physical Activity, Screen Time and Sleep

Laura Stewart

'Doing sport around people who are physically healthier than you can cause a lot of anxiety and it takes a lot of help to get rid of that anxiety'. [1]

Introduction

This is the first of two chapters that focus on the lifestyle behaviour changes recommended in childhood weight management. Guidelines are explicit that childhood weight management programmes should be multicomponent lifestyle interventions that target changes in physical activity, sedentary behaviours and dietary intake [2, 3].

This chapter looks at the hands-on aspects for practitioners in engaging CYP and their families in modifying physical activity and screen time (sedentary behaviours). Sleep and sleep patterns are known to have an association with weight gain and indeed are incorporate into some interventions. Sleep is therefore touched on briefly at the end of this chapter. Dietary modifications are explored in Chapter 7.

Physical Activity

The modern, western, obesogenic environment is considered to encourage a higher usage of screen time and reduced levels of physical activity (PA). Encouraging increased PA should be considered one of the fundamental facets of a childhood multi-component weight management intervention. Increased PA will have a positive effect on energy balance for weight management, instil ongoing healthier behaviours which in turn have health benefits, such as reducing the risk of CVD and type 2 diabetes [2, 4].

Child and Adolescent Obesity: A Practical Approach to Clinical Weight Management,
First Edition. Edited by Laura Stewart.
© 2024 John Wiley & Sons Ltd. Published 2024 by John Wiley & Sons Ltd.

This section on physical activity modification in childhood weight management is aimed at the range of professionals who may work in a weight management service but are not experts in exercise and PA. This section does not aim to explore the physiological aspects of exercise but to discuss the challenges in incorporating PA within clinical programmes, as well as considering how SMART goals could be formulated to encourage an increase in PA for the CYP and their families.

Recommendations on Levels of Physical Activity

There are a number of guidelines around the world which give recommendations on the daily levels of PA for CYP. To cite a few:

- Physical activity guidelines – GOV.UK (www.gov.uk)
- Youth Physical Activity Guidelines|Physical Activity|Healthy Schools|CDC
- Physical activity (who.int)

Both the US (2018) and the UK (2019) guidance on PA levels for CYP recommend that school age CYP should take at least 60 minutes of moderate to vigorous activity (MPVA) per day [5, 6]. The US guidance further breaks this recommendation down into a combination of aerobic type activity, muscle strengthening activities, and bone strengthening activities for at least three days per week [5].

What Does this Mean?

Moderate to Vigorous Activity

The intensity of the level of PA is important in terms of the level of energy expended by the body. MVPA is one way used to describe the intensity of activity undertaken. MVPA will often be seen in the literature in terms of metabolic equivalents (METs), with 3–<6 METS moderate and >6 METs vigorous activity [7]. One MET is described by the WHO as *the energy expended by an individual while seated at rest* [8]. Work around exercise and energy expenditure suggests that resting energy expenditure varies between people and is considered lower for people living with obesity [9].

Another way that levels of PA will frequently be reported in research papers is by the wearing of and then analysis of accelerometers. Accelerometers could be described as a sophisticated form of a step counter; they are typically worn on the waist and record movement. The data can then be downloaded and analysed to give a picture of the amount of time spent in MVPA, light activity and sedentary time [10].

In practice weight management clinics, do not commonly record PA in METs or by using accelerometers. The objective from a weight management perspective is to get the CYP moving, while helping them explore activities that they will find fun and could be incorporated into their daily/weekly routines. In terms of examples, moderate activity would be walking or dancing. Whereas vigorous intensity activity would include jogging, running, brisk walking, cycling or swimming [7]. The language used to describe the different levels of PA to CYP and their families is important, an effective and easy to understand way is to talk about 'getting hot, sweaty and red in the face'.

Aerobic Activity

Aerobic is the term used to describe PA which will increase the heart rate as the body 'uses oxygen', often called cardio fitness. This would include brisk walking, jogging or swimming.

Muscle Strengthening

Muscle strengthening activities involve repetitive movements of muscle group/s, often with a level of resistance such as lifting weights, elastic band type resistance or even press ups.

Bone Strengthening

Bone strengthening exercises are those which involve weight bearing, particularly with some form of 'impact'. These could be running, climbing, jumping or star jumps type activities, and using skipping ropes.

In reality, research has found that most CYP do not regularly meet the national recommendation of at least 60 minutes of physical activity a day [11]. One study suggested that 41% of CYP, aged 10–11 years, in the UK are failing to meet this target [12]. Studies reporting on levels of PA for CYP consistently report that boys spend more time being active than girls [13]. Levels of PA are also reported to decrease and sedentary time increase, for both boys and girls, through adolescence [14]. A number of UK studies, using accelerometer data, showed that total time spent on PA, for both boys and girls, starts to reduce by age 6 to 7 years [15, 16]. Emerging evidence is showing that PA levels for CYP reduced during COVID-19 lockdowns and appears not to have returned to pre-lockdown levels. Salway et al. reported a reduction of 7-8 minutes of MVPA per day for CYP post COVID-19 in the UK [12].

Supporting Increasing Physical Activity Levels in Weight Management Interventions

While any member of a weight management team might help set goals around increasing PA with a CYP and their family, it is crucial that only a suitably qualified professional actually delivers PA sessions or gives specific exercise advice. For example, a physiotherapist in an MDT or a trained exercise instructor from a partner organisation.

When encouraging increased PA levels with CYP living with obesity, particularly those with extreme levels of excess weight, thought should be given to:

- Joint Pain – for example low impact activities may be more suitable such as swimming and cycling.
- Breathlessness – slowly building up activity time and intensity is suitable for everyone.
- Age-appropriate activities – for pre-school children the aim is for them to be running around, playing in the park or garden, spending less time in a pram and walking. While for older children, and in particular adolescents, there may be more consideration of structured and team type activities.
- CYP with additional needs, including those who are wheelchair bound – specialist knowledge is needed to adopt PA to specific needs. The UK's Chief Medical Officers (CMOs) give specific advice around recommendations, see – <u>UK Chief Medical Officers' physical activity guidelines for disabled children and disabled young people: infographic</u> (publishing.service.gov.uk).

If there is any doubt on the type of activities to be recommended to any age of CYP living with obesity, then expert exercise and activity advice should be sought.

In practice, many CYP seen in a weight management clinic will be starting at low level of PA. The reasons will be multiple and for many will include the stigma that they may have been subjected to while taking part in 'exercise'. For example, many will have felt embarrassed, perhaps from negative comments while getting changed into gym clothes in communal changing areas for school physical education (PE). Some will have felt uncomfortable taking part in running sports which may have led to breathlessness and discomfort [17].

Even the word *'exercise'* can have negative connotations for many CYP living with obesity and it is preferable for practitioners to talk about *'being active'*, *'activity'* and *'physical activity levels'*. It is not unheard of to meet some young people who have become school 'avoiders' over the stigma and embarrassment they have experienced during school PE. It is therefore important for the weight management team to encourage and support increasing PA levels in a non-threatening manner and in what feels like a safe environment to the CYP.

While 60 minutes of daily PA is a recommendation for all school aged CYP [5, 6], it is important to work towards this incrementally by setting SMART goals. For example, an initial SMART goal could be – *'To have at least 20 minutes of activity on 2 days each week, until the next session.'* The PA time could be split up over a day into blocks of 10 minutes. Setting such small, but achievable, goals can increase the likelihood of achieving the goal, thus giving a sense of ability and confidence around PA [2].

Structured Versus Daily Activities

When setting goals on increasing physical activity with CYP and their parents, consider the differences between structured, organised activity such as football, swimming and dancing classes and daily activities such as walking, playing in the park, cycling and taking the stairs [2, 6]. For those with very low levels of PA and a perceived dislike of structured PA, a first SMART goal may look like – *'To walk home from school two days next week.'* A stretched SMART goal would be *'To walk home from school at least three days next week.'*

PA Delivery Mode

In group-based childhood weight management programmes, there is typically a section of activities for the CYP within this group environment. The MEND (Mind, Exercise, Nutrition, Do It) programme is one such group-based family weight management programme which incorporates activity sessions into the programme [18, 19]. The sessions are based on demonstrating that being active can be fun. While structured they include activities such as running around, touching base at coloured hoops and collecting bean bags.

It is more of a challenge incorporating PA sessions into a programme that delivered one-to-one. Often the PA will be offered through local leisure centre groups or third sector/charity activity groups, e.g. a local young person's walking group. Virtual PA sessions are also a possible way to encourage weekly PA. In this scenario, some of the considerations for the service will include:-

- Appropriate age group activities are being offered
- Types of activities being offered

- Who is invited to the sessions, e.g. CYP referred to service only or the CYP and their parent or the CYP and family members
- Individual or group physical activity sessions
- Free to families or a small charge to be made
- How the PA is funded
- Local service level agreements (SLAs) with a partner organisation.

There are many ways in which this type of PA support can be offered to CYP and their families. One such way is discussed in a case study in Chapter 11. For CYP with extreme level BMIs, they may require more specialist support to start increasing activity levels such as the input of a paediatric physiotherapist.

Sedentary Behaviours

Sedentary behaviours are defined as time spent being inactive while awake, they habitually involve sitting or lying down [20]. Much of the early work looking at sedentary behaviours and childhood obesity revolved around television (TV) watching [21–23]. As early as 1985, Dietz and Gortmaker from the US described an association, particularly in adolescents, of the time watching TV and obesity [21]. There were two main arguments put forward to explain this association, first that the time spent viewing TV displaced the amount of time during the day to take part in PA. Second, that the viewing of TV was a behavioural antecedent to eating high sugar/high fat energy dense snacks. While the advertising of high energy foods on TV was a further prompt for the intake of high energy dense snacks [3, 21, 24, 25].

Research, mainly from the US-based Epstein group, showed that targeting sedentary behaviours, in particularly TV viewing, could lead to a significant reduction in overweight in CYP. This body of work showed that targeting sedentary behaviours could lead to increased PA levels and was more effective in supporting CYP make long-term changes to their activity rather than targeting PA alone [26, 27]. A number of more up-to-date reviews looking at effects of screen time on CYP report that high screen time is not only associated with weight gain but also with low mood, cognitive and socio-emotional development and educational performance [20, 28–30].

Time Spent on Screens

The term 'screen time' is often used in childhood weight management programmes rather than just targeting TV viewing. This in large is due to the increased usage of other types of screen-based appliances by CYP, such as laptops, mobile phones and tablets. Salway et al. commenting on changes in the types of screen used reported a reduction in TV viewing while at the same time an increase in other types of screen usage [31]. Total time spent on screens by CYP has also been reported as increasing, for example in the US it has increased by 32% over the last 20 years [31, 32]. This increased usage of computers, mobile phone and tablets has added to concerns about the inactive time spent on screens and led to an emphasis on reducing screen time for all CYP.

In the UK, it was reported that in 2019, CYP aged 8–11 year olds spent 5.4 hours per day on screens [31]. This screen time was identified as a combination of watching TV, YouTube, social media and gaming usage [33]. Salway et al. reported that boys spend more of their time than girls on screens, typically on gaming. Also that CYP from lower SES groups tend to have higher screen time [31]. A 2023 study from the International Children Accelerometery Database (ICAD) showed that both boys and girls spent around 6 hours per day on sedentary behaviours [13]. One review has reported that 65–90% of waking time, equivalent to 10 hours per day, are being spent in sedentary behaviours [11]. A survey carried out by the Royal College of Paediatricians and Child Health (RCPCH) showed that the average daily time spent on screens by CYP in the UK was broken down into

- 2.5 hours on computers, laptops and tablets
- 3 hours on phones
- 2 hours on TV viewing [34].

There is no doubt that during COVID-19 lockdowns and school closures, the time spent on screens increased for CYP. Studies are emerging that suggest sustained increases in the time CYP spend on screens post COVID-19 lockdowns [31]. Salway et al. showed, in the UK, an increase in screen time post lockdown of around 30 minutes on week days and 15 minutes during the weekend [12].

Recommendations on Levels of Screen Time

The WHO guidance strongly recommends that sedentary time should be limited for CYP aged 5–17 years old, particularly the amount of 'recreational' screen time [35, 36]. The US guidance on PA for Americans discussed the importance for improving health outcomes of the population by reducing all sedentary time but did not set any recommended time limits for CYP or adults [5]. The Canadian Paediatric Society recommended minimising screen time and reducing risks associated with CYP watching screens [30].

In the UK, the RCPCH recommended taking an individualised approach with parents negotiating screen time limits with their children. Their report acknowledged that there is no defined safe level of screen time for CYP [34]. Having reviewed the evidence on this topic, the RCPCH developed a helpful information sheets for professionals and parents/carers (The health impacts of screen time – a guide for clinicians and parents|RCPCH).

For children under 5 years, the WHO (2019) recommends the following:-

- *'Infants (less than 1 year)* should not be restrained for more than 1 hour at a time (e.g. in prams/strollers, high chairs, or strapped on a caregiver's back). Screen time is not recommended. When sedentary, engaging in reading and storytelling with a caregiver is encouraged.*
- *Children 1–2 years of age* should not be restrained for more than 1 hour at a time (e.g. in prams/strollers, high chairs, or strapped on a caregiver's back) or sit for extended periods of time. For 1-year olds, sedentary screen time (such as watching TV or videos, playing computer games) is not recommended. For those aged 2 years, sedentary screen time should be no more than 1 hour; less is better. When sedentary, engaging in reading and storytelling with a caregiver is encouraged.*
- *Children 3–4 years of age* should not be restrained for more than 1 hour at a time (e.g. in prams/strollers) or sit for extended periods of time. Sedentary screen time should be no more than 1 hour; less is better. When sedentary, engaging in reading and storytelling with a caregiver is encouraged.' [8].*

Supporting Reducing Screen Time in Weight Management Interventions

The early work by the Epstein group recommended that time spent watching TV, playing on computers and video games should be no more than 2 hours a day or 14 hours a week [26, 27]. More recent reviews around screen time and obesity have reported a 42% higher risk of developing childhood overweight or obesity when greater than two hours per day is spent on watching TV compared to two or less hours of viewing [3].

The current practice in childhood weight management clinics is to take the pragmatic approach by first establishing the current typical amount of time spent on all screens and then supporting the CYP to work towards reducing that total time through SMART goals. For many CYP being able to reduce their screen time can be exceedingly challenging. Initial possible SMART goals might look like *'To spend no more than six hours on screen time for two days each week'* or *'No screens to be used after 9pm on two days a week'*. With stretching these goals to *'To spend no more than six hours on screen time for four days each week'* or *'No screens to be used after 9pm on three days a week'*.

Sleep

Sleep is not always seen as a targeted change in childhood weight management programmes. However, targeting improved sleep quality is part of sufficient programmes to warrant discussion in this chapter. It tends to be a component of programmes aimed at younger children or when the programme's outcomes are more focused on healthier lifestyle behaviours rather than on weight and BMI.

There is good evidence to suggest that both the length and timing of sleep patterns can affect energy balance and thus influence weight gain. Studies have identified a relationship between short sleep duration, metabolic disturbances and weight gain. Although the exact mechanisms are still unclear, research suggests that reduced and disturbed sleep may negatively influence the hormones that regulate appetite, in particular insulin, ghrelin and leptin. While disturbed sleep patterns are in turn thought to influence weight gain by tiredness during the day reducing PA time, increasing both night time usage of screens and night time snacking [3, 8, 37–39].

Great Ormond St Hospital in London, UK, recommend the following of good quality sleep times for CYP: 11–14 hours (including day time naps) for 1–2 year olds; 10–13 hours for 3–5 year olds; 9–11 hours for 6–13 year olds; and 8–10 hours for teenagers [40].

A number of studies have demonstrated that reduced sleep duration for younger children increases the risk of developing obesity [41–43]. A 2015 systematic review, demonstrated that children with less than 10 hours of sleep were 76% more likely to have overweight/obesity compared to those with more than 12 hours of sleep a night. Interestingly, they reported that an increase of sleep time by each 1 hour unit per night saw a reduction of the risk overweight/obesity of 21% (OR: 0.79; 95% CI: 0.70, 0.89) [44].

Sleep is determined by the body's circadian rhythm with this influenced by light/darkness and the hormones melatonin and cortisol [45]. It is worth practitioners being aware that adolescents going through puberty see a change in their production of melatonin and cortisol which affects their sleep's circadian rhythm and naturally programmes them to go to sleep and wake up later [45]. This makes week day routines for school naturally difficult for them and disturbs their sleep pattern [8, 46]. Sleep length and quality for adolescents is picked up again in Chapter 12.

Supporting Sleep Quality in Weight Management

Targeting sleep as part of a weight management programme is around supporting improvements in the quality of the CYP's sleep. Sleep hygiene is the term that is generally given to a regular bedtime routine.

Sleep Hygiene

Bedtime routines and timing will differ from young children to adolescents but the overall concept of a regular routine to help settle at bedtime is the same.

Typically, recommendations for good sleep hygiene and improved quality of sleep include:-

- Having a regular (and age appropriate) time to go to bed
- Have a quiet period before bed time
- Taking a bath
- Brushing teeth
- Avoiding sugary and/or caffeinated drinks before bedtime
- Getting into pyjamas
- Having a comfort toy or blanket (for younger children)
- Turning off computers, TV screens, phones, and all screens
- Reading a book or for younger children having a book being read to them.

The bedroom environment is also important for falling asleep and avoiding an interrupted night's sleep. Suggestions could include using black out blinds/curtains in the bedroom, ensuring that the room is not too hot, making it a quiet room with little noise. For younger children that are wary of the dark using a nightlight.

Typical goals around improving sleep quality could be *'Starting the bedtime routine of having a bath, changing into PJs and have a story read at 7pm for three nights next week'* or *'Not having the mobile phone in the bedroom for two nights until the next session'*. Stretched goals could then be *'Starting the bedtime routine of having a bath, changing into PJs and have a story read at 7pm for Monday to Friday nights next week'* or *'Not having the mobile phone in the bedroom for three nights until the next session.'*

While the information above will be appropriate for most CYP attending weight management, there will be some CYP that require further and more expert advice. When sleep patterns are extremely disturbed, the weight management practitioner may need to consider referral of the family to a specialist service. Many sleep specialist services are found in the third sector and have a wealth of experience in giving advice and ongoing support to parents. CYP who are suspected of suffering from sleep apnoea should be referred to an appropriate paediatric specialist.

WHAT DOES THIS MEAN FOR PRACTICE?

Changes to lifestyle behaviours around PA, screen time and sleep quality are important aspects of multi-component CYP's weight management programmes. Changes in all three of these areas should be facilitated through using SMART goals that are realistic for the CYP and their parents to implement.

Increasing PA levels should include every day activities such as walking instead of using the car or bus as well as supporting the CYP to discover 'fun' activities that they feel comfortable taking part in.

Screen time should consider all types of screens used for recreation including mobile phone, computers, game consoles and tablets. While there are some WHO and national guidance around the amount of time CYP spend on screens, negotiating with them small, stepped reduction is a realistic and achievable approach to take.

Targeting improving sleep quality is used as a component in some CYP weight management programmes. Supporting good sleep hygiene involves helping the parents and CYP develop both a quiet period before bed and a regular bedtime routine.

References

1 Rigby, E., McKoewn, R., and Wortley, L. (2022). The experiences of young people and their families living with excess weight: themes from engagement work. https://ayph.org.uk/wp-content/uploads/2022/04/CEW-Themes-from-engagement-work.pdf (accessed 11 May 2024).
2 NICE (2023). Obesity: identification, assessment and management.
3 Hampl, S.E., Hassink, S.G., Skinner, A.C. et al. (2023). Clinical practice guideline for the evaluation and treatment of children and adolescents with obesity. *Pediatrics* 151: e2022060640. https://doi.org/10.1542/peds.2022-060640.
4 Brandt, C. and Pedersen, B.K. (2022). Physical activity, obesity and weight loss maintenance. *Handb. Exp. Pharmacol.* 274: 349–369. https://doi.org/10.1007/164_2021_575.
5 U.S. Department of Health and Human Services *Physical Activity Guidelines for Americans*. Washington, DC: U.S. Department of Health and Human Services. http://doi.org.10.1249/fit.0000000000000472.

6 UK Chief Medical Officers UK Chief Medical Officers' Physical Activity Guidelines. UK Chief Medical Officers 2019 1–65. https://www.gov.uk/government/publications/physical-activity-guidelines-uk-chief-medical-officers-report

7 MacIntosh, B.R., Murias, J.M., Keir, D.A. et al. (2021). What is moderate to vigorous exercise intensity? *Front. Physiol.* 12: 682233. https://doi.org/10.3389/fphys.2021.682233.

8 World Health Organization (2019). *WHO Guideline: Physical Activity, Sedentary Behavior and Sleep for Children under 5 Years of Age.* Geneva: World Health Organization. http://doi.org/10.1055/a-1489-8049.

9 Franklin, B.A., Brinks, J., Berra, K. et al. (2018). Using metabolic equivalents in clinical practice. *Am. J. Cardiol.* 121: 382–387. https://doi.org/10.1016/j.amjcard.2017.10.033.

10 Lee, I.M. and Shiroma, E.J. (2014). Using accelerometers to measure physical activity in large scale epidemiological studies: Issues and challenges. *Br. J. Sports Med.* 48: 197–201. https://doi.org/10.1136/bjsports-2013-093154.

11 Elmesmari, R., Martin, A., Reilly, J.J. et al. (2018). Comparison of accelerometer measured levels of physical activity and sedentary time between obese and non-obese children and adolescents: a systematic review. *BMC Pediatr.* 18: https://doi.org/10.1186/s12887-018-1031-0.

12 Salway, R., Foster, C., de Vocht, F. et al. (2022). Accelerometer-measured physical activity and sedentary time among children and their parents in the UK before and after COVID-19 lockdowns: a natural experiment. *Int. J. Behav. Nutr. Phys. Act.* 19: 51. https://doi.org/10.1186/s12966-022-01290-4.

13 Kretschmer, L., Salali, G.D., Andersen, L.B. et al. (2023). Gender differences in the distribution of children's physical activity: evidence from nine countries. *Int. J. Behav. Nutr. Phys. Act.* 20: 1–10. https://doi.org/10.1186/s12966-023-01496-0.

14 Cooper, A.R., Goodman, A., Page, A.S. et al. (2015). Objectively measured physical activity and sedentary time in youth: the International children's accelerometry database (ICAD). *Int. J. Behav. Nutr. Phys. Act.* 12: 1–10. https://doi.org/10.1186/s12966-015-0274-5.

15 Farooq, M.A., Parkinson, K.N., Adamson, A.J. et al. (2018). Timing of the decline in physical activity in childhood and adolescence: Gateshead Millennium Cohort Study. *Br. J. Sports Med.* 52: 1002–1006. https://doi.org/10.1136/bjsports-2016-096933.

16 Jago, R., Salway, R., Emm-Collison, L. et al. (2020). Association of BMI category with change in children's physical activity between ages 6 and 11 years: a longitudinal study. *Int. J. Obes.* 44: 104–113. https://doi.org/10.1038/s41366-019-0459-0.

17 Shim, Y.M., Burnette, A., Lucas, S. et al. (2013). Physical deconditioning as a cause of breathlessness among obese adolescents with a diagnosis of asthma. *PLoS One* 8: 1–7. https://doi.org/10.1371/journal.pone.0061022.

18 Sacher, P.M., Kolotourou, M., Chadwick, P.M. et al. (2010). Randomized controlled trial of the MEND program: a family-based community

intervention for childhood obesty. *Obesity* 18: S62–S68. https://doi.org/10.1038/oby.2009.433.

19 Liu, S., Weismiller, J., Strange, K. et al. (2020). Evaluation of the scale-up and implementation of mind, exercise, nutrition … do it! (MEND) in British Columbia: a hybrid trial type 3 evaluation. *BMC Pediatr.* 20: 1–11. https://doi.org/10.1186/s12887-020-02297-1.

20 Tremblay, M.S., Aubert, S., Barnes, J.D. et al. (2017). SBRN Terminology Consensus Project Participants. Sedentary Behavior Research Network (SBRN) – Terminology Consensus Project process and outcome. *Int. J. Behav. Nutr. Phys. Act* 14 (1): 75. (accessed 11 May 2024).

21 Dietz, W.H. and Gortmaker, S.L. (1985). Do we fatten our children at the television set? Obesity and television viewing in children and adolescents. *Pediatrics* 75: 807 LP–812 LP. http://pediatrics.aappublications.org/content/75/5/807.abstract.

22 Ludwig, D.S. and Gortmaker, S.L. (2004). Programming obesity in childhood. *Lancet* 364: 226–227. https://doi.org/10.1016/S0140-6736(04)16688-9.

23 Gortmaker, S.L., Must, A., Sobol, A.M. et al. (1996). Television viewing as a cause of increasing obesity among children in the United States, 1986–1990. *Arch. Pediatr. Adolesc. Med.* 150: 356–362. https://doi.org/10.1001/archpedi.1996.02170290022003.

24 Wiecha, J.L., Peterson, K.E., Ludwig, D.S. et al. (2006). When children eat what they watch: impact of television viewing on dietary intake in youth. *Arch. Pediatr. Adolesc. Med.* 160: 436–442. https://doi.org/10.1001/archpedi.160.4.436.

25 Lobstein, T. and Dibb, S. (2005). Evidence of a possible link between obesogenic food advertising and child overweight. *Obes. Rev.* 6: 203–208. https://doi.org/10.1111/j.1467-789X.2005.00191.x.

26 Epstein, L.H., Valoski, A.M., Vara, L.S. et al. (1995). Effects of decreasing sedentary behavior and increasing activity on weight change in obese children. *Heal. Psychol.* 14: 109–115. https://doi.org/10.1037/0278-6133.14.2.109.

27 Epstein, L.H., Paluch, R.A., Gordy, C.C. et al. (2000). Problem solving in the treatment of childhood obesity. *J. Consult. Clin. Psychol.* 68: 717–721. https://doi.org/10.1037/0022-006X.68.4.717.

28 Stiglic, N. and Viner, R.M. (2019). Effects of screentime on the health and well-being of children and adolescents: A systematic review of reviews. *BMJ Open.* 9: https://doi.org/10.1136/bmjopen-2018-023191.

29 Davies, S.C., Atherton, F., and Calderwood, C. et al. (2019). United Kingdom Chief Medical Officers' commentary on 'Screen-based activities and children and young people's mental health and psychosocial wellbeing:a systematic map of reviews'.

30 Canadian Paediatric Society DHTF (2017). Screen time and young children: Promoting health and development in a digital world. *Paediatr. Child. Heal.* 22: 461–477. https://doi.org/10.1093/pch/pxx123.

31 Salway, R., Walker, R., Sansum, K. et al. (2023). Screen-viewing behaviours of children before and after the 2020–21 COVID-19 lockdowns in the UK: a mixed methods study. *BMC Publ. Health* 23: 1–14. https://doi.org/10.1186/s12889-023-14976-6.

32 Bergmann, C., Dimitrova, N., Alaslani, K. et al. (2022). Young children's screen time during the first COVID-19 lockdown in 12 countries. *Sci. Rep.* 12: 1–15. https://doi.org/10.1038/s41598-022-05840-5.

33 OfCom (2020/21). Children and Parents: Media Use and Attitudes Report. 2021. https://www.ofcom.org.uk/__data/assets/pdf_file/0025/217825/children-and-parents-media-use-and-attitudes-report-2020-21.pdf (accessed 11 May 2024).

34 Royal College of Paediatrics and Child Health (2019). The health impacts of screen time: a guide for clinicians and parents.https://www.rcpch.ac.uk/sites/default/files/2018-12/rcpch_screen_time_guide_-_final.pdf (accessed 02 September 2023).

35 Bull, F.C., Al-Ansari, S.S., Biddle, S. et al. (2020). World Health Organization 2020 guidelines on physical activity and sedentary behaviour. *Br. J. Sports Med.* 54: 1451–1462. https://doi.org/10.1136/bjsports-2020-102955.

36 WHO (2020). *WHO Guidelines on Physical Activity and Sedentary Behaviour*. Geneva: World Health Organization. https://www.ncbi.nlm.nih.gov/books/NBK566045/pdf/Bookshelf_NBK566045.pdf.

37 Taheri, S. (2006). The link between short sleep duration and obesity. *Arch. Dis. Child.* 91: 881–884. https://doi.org/10.1136/adc.2005.093013.

38 Skjåkødegård, H.F., Danielsen, Y.S., Frisk, B. et al. (2021). Beyond sleep duration: sleep timing as a risk factor for childhood obesity. *Pediatr. Obes.* 16: 1–11. https://doi.org/10.1111/ijpo.12698.

39 Chaput, J.-P. (2014). Sleep patterns, diet quality and energy balance. *Physiol. Behav.* 134: 86–91. https://doi.org/10.1016/j.physbeh.2013.09.006.

40 Great Ormand St. Hospital *Paediatric Sleep. Helping Your Child Get a Good Night's Sleep*. London: Great Ormand St. Hospital. https://media.gosh.nhs.uk/documents/GOSH_Sleep_Hygiene_in_children.pdf.

41 Reilly, J.J. and Hughes, A.R. (2015). Early life risk factors for childhood obesity. In: *Early Years Nutrition and Healthy Weight* (ed. L. Stewart and J. Thompson), 40–45. Wiley.

42 Fatima Y, Doi SAR, Mamun AA. Longitudinal impact of sleep on overweight and obesity in children and adolescents: a systematic review and bias-adjusted meta-analysis. *Obes. Rev.* 2015;16:137–49. https://doi.org/10.1111/obr.12245

43 Morrissey, B., Taveras, E., Allender, S. et al. (2020). Sleep and obesity among children: a systematic review of multiple sleep dimensions. *Pediatr. Obes.* 15: 1–21. https://doi.org/10.1111/ijpo.12619.

44 Ruan, H., Xun, P., Cai, W. et al. (2015). Habitual sleep duration and risk of childhood obesity: systematic review and dose-response meta-analysis of prospective cohort studies. *Sci. Rep.* 5: 1–14. https://doi.org/10.1038/srep16160.

45 National Research Council and Institute of Medicine (2000). *Sleep Needs, Patterns, and Difficulties of Adolescents. Forum on Adolescence*. Washington, D.C: National Research Council and Institute of Medicine. https://www.ncbi.nlm.nih.gov/books/NBK222800/pdf/Bookshelf_NBK222800.pdf.

46 Morales-Ghinaglia, N. and Fernandez-Mendoza, J. (2023). Sleep variability and regularity as contributors to obesity and cardiometabolic health in adolescence. *Obesity (Silver Spring)* 31: 597–614. https://doi.org/10.1002/oby.23667.

7 Modifying Energy Intake

Laura Stewart

'It takes time and a lot of hard work'. [1]

Introduction

Chapter 6 looked at one side of the energy balance by exploring modifying physical activity levels and screen time. This chapter takes the next step in considering energy balance by examining ways to modify and reduce the energy intake, which will always be the key element of childhood weight management [2, 3]. While most of the dietary changes a CYP and their family will undertake will be guided by a dietitian, it is important that others in the team are aware of the possible types of dietary modifications that might be recommended and the evidence base/good practice that sits behind the strategies employed.

An important facet of managing weight in childhood is that CYP are still growing and their body is developing. Therefore, it is essential to ensure that age-appropriate amounts of protein, vitamins and minerals are within any energy modification. Before looking at strategies for energy modification to CYP's intake, it is worth spending a short time considering a balanced nutritional intake in childhood and adolescence.

Balanced Nutritional Intake

To achieve optimal growth and maintain good health throughout childhood and adolescence, a well-balanced dietary intake is paramount. An optimal average daily intake of energy, protein, carbohydrates, fats, vitamins and minerals is essential.

Child and Adolescent Obesity: A Practical Approach to Clinical Weight Management,
First Edition. Edited by Laura Stewart.
© 2024 John Wiley & Sons Ltd. Published 2024 by John Wiley & Sons Ltd.

Discussed later in Chapter 9 on the early years, it is accepted that breastfeeding from birth has a number of on-going health benefits [4, 5]. Breast milk contains all the necessary nutrients for optimal growth in new born children. The WHO recommends that breastfeeding (or formula milks) is the sole source of nutrition until around six months of age when solid foods can start to be introduced [6]. This is known to many people as 'weaning' but now tends to be called complementary feeding. The WHO described this period as –

> 'Complementary feeding, defined as the process of providing foods in addition to milk when breast milk or milk formula alone are no longer adequate to meet nutritional requirements, generally starts at age 6 months and continues until 23 months of age. This is a developmental period when it is critical for children to learn to accept healthy foods and beverages and establish long-term dietary patterns' [6].

During this time, young children's intake of solid foods increase, while the reliance on milk gradually decreases. They move towards establishing an eating pattern that is similar to the family with typically three meals per day – breakfast, lunch and evening meal, as well as typically two to three snacks per day. Guidance on the types of foods, portion sizes and timings of feeding will vary between country and regions; however, most will be based around the advice from the WHO of introducing complementary feeding at around six months [6]. It would be good practice to have an understanding of the local and national policy on complementary feeding guidance.

Across the globe, there are a variety of graphic models that illustrate what constitutes a healthy balance diet for that population. The Food and Agriculture Organization of the UN (FAO) gives very insightful background information about dietary guidelines and the ways in which they have been developed and used in different countries and regions (see Background|Food-based dietary guidelines|Food and Agriculture Organization of the United Nations (fao.org)). The following links give examples of graphic illustrations of national guidance on a healthy balanced dietary intake -

- The Eatwell Guide (publishing.service.gov.uk)
- USDA MyPlate What Is MyPlate?
- Healthy Eating Pyramid|Nutrition Australia.

The next section explores modification of energy intake for CYP, while being mindful of the need for age-appropriate intakes of essential nutrients.

Energy Modification Strategies

It is always worth remembering that all foods and drinks – except water – contain energy that can be either utilised or stored by the human body. Therefore, in weight management it is important that all sources of energy intake are considered when looking to reduce total energy intake (TEI). While aiming to reduce TEI, a number of different food group/food types have been emphasised as potentially making the greatest impact for weight management in CYP [2, 7], some of these are explored below as well as snacking, beverages and age-appropriate portion sizes.

A systematic review of dietary modifications for childhood weight management made the following recommendations in a report to the WHO:

1. *'Monitoring of dietary intake by child, parent or adolescent using a dietary intake monitoring tool, such as a food diary or diet application.*
2. *Self or family-led self-evaluation using comparison of collected dietary intake with recommendations in dietary guidelines.*
3. *Strategies that targeted specific dietary components, e.g. strategies to decrease SSB (sugar-sweetened drinks) or EDNP (energy dense, nutrient poor) intake, rather than more general healthy eating advice.*
4. *Strategies that prioritise personalised behaviour change based on individual health education or behaviour needs.*
5. *Use of health coaching techniques by health professionals to assist individuals to identify, prioritise, implement and evaluate agreed, prioritised health behaviour changes'* [7].

It is important while working within a standardised programme to ensure that the actual lifestyle, including dietary, changes are individualised to the particular CYP and their family situation [2]. It is therefore a good place to start by asking the family and CYP to monitor their own intake using a lifestyle diary. This is a good starting place to explore patterns of meals, snacks and drinks. While, during in person discussions, to use a person-friendly 'typical day', understanding when food, drink, physical activity and screen time sit within a typical day for the CYP. This exploring will always be a process which continues over the sessions of the programme [8].

A Traffic Light Scheme

A 2012 systematic review, by Ho et al., look at energy modification strategies that had been deployed in weight management research programmes across the world [9]. This review found that the most frequently used approach was a 'traffic light' dietary scheme. This traffic light concept originates from work in the US over a number of years from Leonard Epstein's team [10].

A traffic light scheme allocates food and drinks depending on their energy density to red, amber or green categories. Typically, red foods are high-energy-type snacks and fast foods, amber foods are moderate energy including non-fried protein and carbohydrates and green are low-energy dense foods such as fruit and vegetables. The energy intake is modified through highlighting the need to cut back on red foods, eat a moderate amount of the amber foods, while green foods can be freely taken and swapped for the higher energy red foods [9, 11].

Epstein original traffic light scheme was complex with an aim of an energy restriction of circa 1200 kcal/day. Green foods had an energy value less than 20 kcal per average portion. Amber foods were categorised in the four basic food groups and energy restricted. Red foods had an energy restriction of being not over 300 kcal per serving, plus in an attempt to change people's food preferences, low-fat alternatives e.g. low-fat lasagna was also categorised as red. The aim was to limit red foods to four to seven portions per week [12].

Other programmes have taken the basic structure of a traffic light dietary scheme and made it less complex. A less strict manner in which to use the traffic light dietary scheme is to consider that:–

- Red foods are stop, be careful, consider how many you need
- Amber are be cautious, particularly of portion sizes
- Green are for go and swapping with red foods [11].

Table 7.1 gives an example of the types of foods and drinks which would sit within each colour category.

Specific Energy Restrictions

Some research studies have targeted a defined dietary energy restriction such as an overall specified energy reduction per day based on current intake or the age-appropriate daily energy requirements [9]. It is more common in clinical practice to see targeting of foods that are particularly high in fat or sugar and thus high in energy.

Many of these high-energy targeted foods come under the umbrella term of 'energy dense, nutrient poor (EDNP) foods'. EDNP foods are those high in sugar and fat while also a poor source of protein, vitamins and minerals.

Table 7.1 Example of a traffic light dietary scheme.

Red Foods	Amber Foods	Green Foods
Fried foods	Lamb, pork, beef	Fresh fruit
Crisps	Chicken and turkey	Dried fruit
Chips (french fries)	Fish	Tinned fruit in fruit juice Vegetables/salad
Pies, pastries, bridies, sausage rolls	Sausages and burgers	Homemade/tinned vegetable soup
Spring rolls, pakoras, samosas, bhajis	Eggs	Sugar-free jelly
Pizza	Cheese	Sugar-free lollies
Carry out meals	Vegetarian and vegan main meals	Water
Fries and burgers	Bread/chapatti	Diet/sugar-free/no added sugar drinks
Chicken nuggets	Potatoes	
Sugar	Boiled rice	
Sweets	Pasta	
Chocolate	Plain breakfast cereals	
Chocolate biscuits		
Fancy biscuits	Low-fat alternatives of –	
Cakes	Milk, butter/margarine	
Sugar-sweetened drinks	Yogurts	
Desserts and puddings		
Cereal bars		
Sugar or honey/chocolate-coated breakfast cereals		

Source: Adapted from Stewart et al. [11].

Typically in a western diet, EDNP foods are sweets, chocolate, cake, biscuits, crisps and salty type snacks [7, 13]. Many of these foods sit under the red category in a traffic light scheme. High sugar-sweetened drinks (SSB) and snacks, while in this category, are dealt with separately below.

From a behavioural and person-centred point of view, EDNP or red category foods should not be described or talked about as 'bad' foods or suggest that they are removed completely from a CYP's intake, instead these are foods and drinks that can be reduced in a considered way through setting person-led behavioural change goals.

Fruits and Vegetables

While most of the dietary modifications discussed have been about reducing intake of a food type, on the other hand, fruits and vegetables are one group that is often actively encouraged to be increased. Fruits and vegetables tend to be lower in energy than EDNP foods and contain essential vitamins and minerals, therefore adding to a balanced nutritional intake. Intakes of fruits and vegetables by CYP tend to be lower than recommendations, for example the 2021 Scottish Health Survey reported that only 20% of CYP age 2–15 years took the recommended five portions per day, with the average number of portions in this age group being 3.4 a day [14].

In practice many parents see increasing fruits and vegetables intake in their children as an up-hill struggle. As with all dietary changes, perseverance and listening to the CYP can make small positive steps. Fruits and vegetables can be successfully used as 'swaps' for higher energy foods/snacks. Modelling of this behaviour, by others in the family, is supportive of the CYP making this change. Most vegetables tend to be lower in energy than fruits so separating the changes can be helpful in impacting on decreasing TEI.

Beverages

Drinks (beverages) can be a significant source of energy intake for both adult and CYP. It is therefore important to remember to gather information regarding both the quantity and types of drinks taken by a CYP. There are a number of different types of drinks which are worth considering at this point.

Sugar-Sweetened Beverages

The first of these drinks to consider are sugar-sweetened beverages (SSBs). The intake of SSBs is recognised as a risk factor in the development of obesity, type 2 diabetes and some cancers in adults [15] and obesity in CYP [16]. They are usually included within the category of EDNP foods but are discussed separately here due to the importance of their association with weight gain.

A 2022 review, by Malik and Hu, on the role of SSB in obesity tells us that currently there is no agreed international definition of what constitutes SSB, they gave a number of qualifications:

> *'The most widely accepted definition used in research is to consider any beverage as an SSB if it contains caloric sweeteners such as sucrose, high- fructose corn syrup (HFCS) or fruit juice concentrates among others, which are added to the beverages by manufacturers, establishments or individuals. However, some authorities have developed more specific definitions based on sugar content per volume, which have been used for regulatory initiatives. For example, the New York City Board of Health defines SSBs as having ≥25 calories or 6.25 g of added sugar per 8 fl oz (~237 ml), whereas in the UK the definition for taxation is ≥5 g of added sugar per 100 ml'* [15].

While a 2019 Cochrane Review defined SSBs as – *'non-alcoholic, non-dairy beverages with added caloric sweeteners. This definition includes, but is not limited to, carbonated soft drinks (sodas), fruit juices with less than 100% fruit content and added sugars, sugar-sweetened energy and sports drinks, sugar-sweetened vitamin waters and flavoured water, and sugar-sweetened coffee and tea beverages. The definition covers both ready-to-drink beverages and beverages prepared by consumers from syrups, concentrates or powder, or by adding sugar to beverages such as tea and coffee'* [17].

SSB intake is an area of dietary and energy intake to explore and discuss with CYP and their families. The most obvious drink to replace SSB with is water; however, in practice a large number of CYP will state that they 'do not like the taste' of water. Other alternatives are drinks, particularly fizzy drinks, with artificial sweeteners. If these are to be suggested/recommended, then it is important to be aware of any regions/countries policy on the use of artificial sweeteners or non-sugar sweeteners (NSS). A WHO 2023 guideline of the use of NSS recommends that they are not use in weight management [18], see – Use of non-sugar sweeteners: WHO guideline.

While juices with sugar replacements may be lower in energy, dentists will still warn against them as the acid in the juice will still affect tooth decay. Another alternative often used by families are flavoured waters; these can be useful however, care needs to be taken as many of these flavoured water drinks also contain sugar.

Milk

While breastfeeding and nutrition in the early years are touched on in Chapter 9, it is appropriate here when discussing beverages as a source of excess energy to consider cow's milk as a drink past one year of age. Certainly, in the UK it is recommended that from one year of age children do not drink more than 500 ml per day of milk. This is because a higher intake of milk can displace other solid foods from the young child's intake; cow's milk also lacks dietary iron.

When seeing pre-school children due to obesity, an excessive intake of milk can be a major dietary factor that needs to be tackled. An approach would be to recommend reducing the volume to 500 ml a day, semi-skimmed milk can be recommended by a health professional for children after two years and fully skimmed milk from five years. If a child older than one is still taking milk from a bottle, then the parents need to be supported to gradually discontinue this habit. This can be an anxious inducing process for parent, particularly if the child is taking milk from a bottle in their cot at night, as they then worry that their child will have a disturbed sleep. A lot of support and a gradual removal is required, for example the milk could be gradually replaced with water, while the bottle could be replaced by an age-appropriate feeding cup. Sugar-sweetened and flavoured milks are not a good alternative for CYP.

Fruit Juice

Fruit juice and smoothies deserve a mention in this section. Pure unsweetened fruit juice is recommended for children under five years as a small glass diluted with water, for example 50 ml fruit juice plus 50 ml water and limited to mealtimes [19].

Smoothies are typically drinks with fruits or vegetables as the base; they are blended and can have for example milk or yoghurt added. While many see these drinks as 'healthy', smoothies can have a high concentration of energy; therefore, it is best to ask parents to read the labels to view the total energy content of a drink.

Table 7.2 gives an overview of the typical energy content of a variety of the drinks that have been discussed in this section.

Snacks

Snacking behaviours are an important point to consider when reviewing CYP's total dietary intake. Many types of snacks taken by CYP will be those high in sugar and fat, with most being categorised as EDNP foods. Therefore, as part of the overall target of decreasing the energy intake, the type and number of snacks is a worthwhile behaviour change to explore [20].

The process of television viewing, has been cited, as encouraging an increased intake of high sugar/high fat energy dense snacks by the behavioural association with eating while watching TV. As discussed in Chapter 6, early research into the association of screen time, mainly TV watching, showed an association with weight gain and obesity [21]. This work has led to the consideration around the interaction of TV watching (screen time) and snacking. Avery et al. showed that there was an association between CYP watching TV and eating foods such as pizza, fried foods and sweets [22]. A further aspect is the influence of TV advertising of high fat/sugar, high-energy snack/fast foods on CYP's choices of foods [23].

Table 7.2 Energy value of typical drinks.

Drink	Kcals/100 ml	Kcals/500 ml	Kcals/1000 ml
Water	0	0	0
Cola	40	200	400
Sugar-free cola	0.3	1.5	3
Fruit juice (orange)	45	225	450
Smoothie	52	260	520
Cow's milk (full fat)	65	325	650
Cow's milk (semi-skimmed)	49	245	490

Averages of a variety of products used for demonstration.

The UK has considered regulations to prohibit advertising of foods high in fat, salt and sugar between 5.30 am and 9 pm (see – New advertising rules to help tackle childhood obesity – GOV.UK (www.gov.uk)).

In practical terms, there are a number of tips that can be recommended to help limit the eating of snacks, such as:–

- Not eating when the television is on
- Only eating food from a plate
- Eating as a family sitting at the table.

The use of a 'snack box' is another strategy which can be successful with CYP. This involves an agreement between the CYP and their parent on the type and number of snacks. These are then placed daily in a box by the parent and the CYP helps themselves as they wish until the snack box is empty. This agreement includes that no other snacks are sought or offered until the next day when the process starts again.

Portion Sizes

When exploring and then modifying energy intake, an important aspect to consider is portion size [24]. We know that, certainly in developed countries, food portion sizes have increased over the last few decades. Research has shown that the portion size seen as normal or typical has increased [25].

It is suggested that consuming larger portions eaten outside the home has influenced overall eating habits and the portions served at home. Particularly the increased portion size seen in 'fast food' restaurants and what has been termed the 'super-size me' portions [26, 27]. Indeed, the manner in which some supermarket and restaurants market the larger sizes have moved consumers towards a 'value for money' frame of mind on portion sizes. Leading to a situation when it can actually cost less to buy larger portions sizes in value packs.

Another tendency towards larger portions in the home is the fashion for large and outsized plates. Research has shown that for both CYP and adults there is a tendency to eat to the size of the plate and spoon used [28].

The reason this blurring of portion size for CYP is important is that offering larger portions sizes to young children can affect the total energy intake. CYP offered larger meal sizes have been shown to both eat a larger amount and take in more total energy. It has been proposed that CYP being given larger portion sizes can start to override their own natural inbuilt feeling of fullness in children as young as two years [29, 30].

From a practical point of view in weight management programmes, practitioners need to explore and consider if age-appropriate portions are being given at meals and for snacks. Many families will not be aware of what are 'normal' age portions and frequently underestimate the portions served in the family home. It is not uncommon to work with families where everyone is served the same portion from the dad to the youngest family member. It is, therefore, very important that practitioners can give the parents a good understanding of what are the correct portion sizes for CYP at different ages. In the UK, there are two main resources around CYP's portion sizes.

- Nutrition and Diet Resources UK (NDR) *Smart Size Portions for Children* (Smart Sized Portions for Children|Nutrition and Diet Resources (ndr-uk.org))
- The Caroline Walker Trust *Eating well for 1–4 year olds. Practical guide* (The Caroline Walker Trust|improving public health through good food (cwt.org.uk))

While in the US, the AAP has produced useful online fact sheets such as – Portions and Serving Sizes – HealthyChildren.org.

During consultations an often useful way to help families understand the differences in suitable age portion sizes is to use the 'handy measures' tools, where:-

- A fist size for carbohydrate/starchy foods
- A palm size for protein foods
- A thumb size for cheese
- A portion of fruit is what can be held in one hand.

This explanation is a very simplified way to help the whole family see the differences in the age-appropriate portion sizes for each family member.

Non-hunger Eating

While this chapter is concerned about energy modification and how this might look in a weight management programme. It is well known that weight management is not as simplistic as eat less do more activity. The 2007 Foresight report demonstrates the complexity and multiple systems that contribute to the aetiology of overweight and obesity [31]. Therefore, it is worth at this point taking a breath and finishing the chapter by considering behaviours and emotions that are associated with eating, which will be a vital part of any clinical conversation in supporting weight management.

It is important in a chapter on modifying energy intake to consider the concepts and aspects of non-hunger eating. As human beings we eat for many reasons not just to take in the nutrients required to keep us fit, healthy and active. Everyone reading this book will be able to relate to eating for various reasons which may be seen as positive such as celebrating a success or birthday or socialising with family and friends. Many also eat from what may be seen as negative cues such as anger, frustration, anxiety or low mood [32]. There is evidence that eating behaviours in people living with obesity becomes dissociated from perceptions of satiety and hunger [33].

When eating behaviours are triggered by the powerful emotions of anxiety and stress, many CYP turn to foods high in sugar and fat – sometimes referred to by people as comfort eating. This can also lead to hiding eating habits. In clinic, parents often talk about finding sweetie wrappers hidden under the young person's bed or even the CYP 'stealing' food from the kitchen. The role of the practitioner working with the family is to understand the eating patterns that are occurring and help the CYP express their feelings and emotions at these times. This can be done by asking the CYP to record their eating patterns alongside the mood and/or the emotional triggers to the non-hunger eating. The majority of these CYP will not require referral to a psychologist, if the practitioner and MDT members have had psychology informed training [32] and are able to use simple tools to help the CYP explore their 'unhelpful thoughts or thinking errors' in an age-appropriate manner. It is important to understand that these triggers can be strong and highly emotional; therefore, discussions with or referral to the psychologist within the MDT or the local service should always be an option for a weight management service.

Another useful tool that practitioners can be trained to use with young people is a hunger score ladder. A hunger score is often used in adult weight management to help people distinguish between points of eating when hungry and not hungry, i.e. recognising non hunger-eating and attempting to work towards reducing it. The same concept can be used with young people using age-appropriate language, such as:–

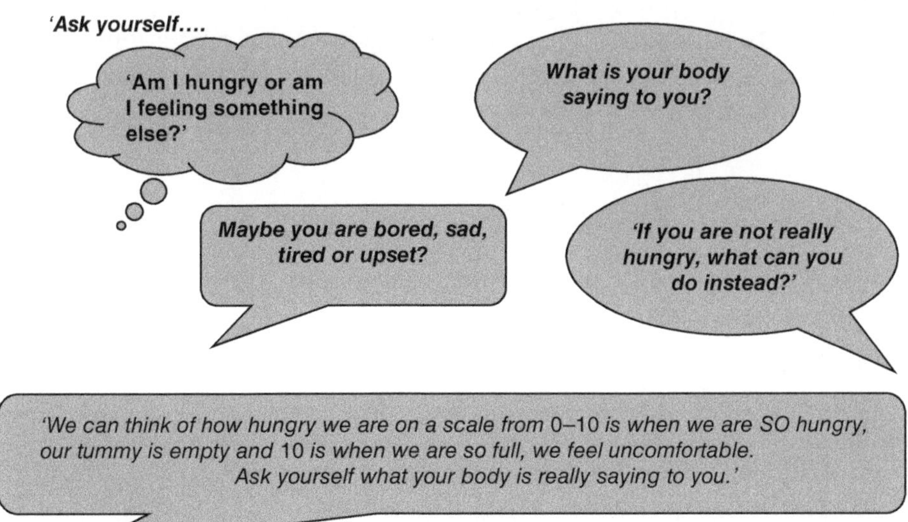

It is important for anyone working in the field of weight management to be able to understand the difference between what is frequently termed, disorder eating and an eating disorder.

*'**Eating disorders** are serious mental illnesses affecting people of all ages, genders, ethnicities and backgrounds. People with eating disorders use disordered eating behaviour as a way to cope with difficult situations or feelings. This behaviour can include limiting the amount of food eaten, eating very large quantities of food at once, getting rid of food eaten through unhealthy means (e.g. making themselves sick, misusing laxatives, fasting, or excessive exercise), or a combination of these behaviours.'* (Types of Eating Disorder (`beateatingdisorders.org.uk`)). Eating disorders (EDs) are diagnosed using the *Diagnostic and Statistical Manual of Mental Disorders* (DSM) classification [34] and include:

- bulimia nervosa
- binge eating disorder (BED)
- avoidant/restrictive food intake disorder (ARFID)
- other specified feeding or eating disorder (OSFED)
- anorexia nervosa.

However, disordered eating is a term that describes eating patterns and behaviours that are not recognised as fitting into regular structured eating. This could range from skipping meals to patterns and behaviours that fall short of the DSM diagnosis classification of an ED. If any practitioner has concerns that a CYP may be exhibiting signs of an eating disorder, these should be discussed with the MDT's psychologist or the local ED team. Further discussion of EDs is outside of the remit of this chapter and book.

Many parents are anxious that their child may develop an ED from taking part in a weight management programme. Whereas a systematic review in 2019 showed that for CYP a *'structured and professionally run obesity treatment was associated with reduced ED prevalence, ED risk, and symptoms'* [35].

WHAT DOES THIS MEAN IN PRACTICE?

When exploring the total energy intake, it is important to look at all possible sources of possible excess energy intake as such:

- EDPN
- Beverages
- Larger portion size for age
- Snacks and snacking behaviours
- For under-fives, milk intake.

All dietary changes within a weight management programme should be individualised to the needs and situation of the CYP and their family. Changes should be considered using behavioural change tools, particularly goal setting and readiness to change.

It is helpful to explore non-hunger eating and to discuss strategies to decrease this behaviour. Any professional in a childhood weight management team should be aware of behaviours which may be a red flag to a possible ED and have a clear agreed pathway for discussing concerns and onward referral.

References

1   Rigby, E., McKoewn, R., and Wortley, L. The experiences of young people and their families living with excess weight: themes from engagement work. https://ayph.org.uk/wp-content/uploads/2022/04/CEW-Themes-from-engagement-work.pdf (accessed 29 March 2024).

2   Duncanson, K., Shrewsbury, V., Burrows, T. et al. (2021). Impact of weight management nutrition interventions on dietary outcomes in children and adolescents with overweight or obesity: a systematic review with meta-analysis. *J. Hum. Nutr. Diet.* 34: 147–177. https://doi.org/10.1111/jhn.12831.

3   Ho, M., Garnett, S.P., Baur, L.A. et al. (2013). Impact of dietary and exercise interventions on weight change and metabolic outcomes in obese children and adolescents. *JAMA Pediatr.* 167: 759. https://doi.org/10.1001/jamapediatrics.2013.1453.

4   World Health Organization (2021). Infant and young child feeding. https://www.who.int/news-room/fact-sheets/detail/infant-and-young-child-feeding (accessed 29 March 2024).

5   SACN (2018). Feeding in the first year of life. https://assets.publishing.service.gov.uk/government/uploads/system/uploads/attachment_data/file/725530/SACN_report_on_Feeding_in_the_First_Year_of_Life.pdf (accessed 29 March 2024).

6   World Health Organization (2023). *WHO Guideline for Complementary Feeding of Infants and Young Children 6–23 Months of Age.* World Health Organization https://www.who.int/publications/i/item/9789240081864.

7   Duncanson, K., Shewbury, V., and Collins, C. et al. (2017). Interim Report on the Effectiveness of Dietary Interventions for Children and Adolescents with Overweight and Obesity Prepared for the World Health Organization Priority Research Centre in Physical Activity and Nutrition. Interim report on the effectiveness of dietary interventions for children and adolescents with overweight and obesity: prepared for the World Health Organization (newcastle.edu.au) (accessed 29 March 2024).

8   Stewart, L., Easter, S., and BDA's Obesity Specialist Group (2021). British Dietetic Association's Obesity Specialist Group dietetic obesity management interventions in children and young people: review & clinical application. *J. Hum. Nutr. Diet.* 34: 224–232. https://doi.org/10.1111/jhn.12834.

9 Ho, M., Garnett, S.P., Baur, L. et al. (2012). Effectiveness of lifestyle interventions in child obesity: systematic review with meta-analysis. *Pediatrics* 130: https://doi.org/10.1542/peds.2012-1176.

10 Epstein, L.H., Valoski, A., Wing, R.R. et al. (1994). Ten-year outcomes of behavioral family-based treatment for childhood obesity. *Health Psychol.* 13: 373–383. https://doi.org/10.1037/0278-6133.13.5.373.

11 Stewart, L., Houghton, J., Hughes, A.R. et al. (2005). Dietetic management of pediatric overweight: development and description of a practical and evidence-based behavioral approach. *J. Am. Diet. Assoc.* 105: 1810–1815. https://doi.org/10.1016/j.jada.2005.08.006.

12 Epstein, L.H., Wing, R.R., and Valoski, A. (1985). Childhood obesity. *Pediatr. Clin. N. Am.* 32: 363–379. https://doi.org/10.1016/S0031-3955(16)34792-7.

13 Biltoft-Jensen, A., Matthiessen, J., Hess Ygil, K. et al. (2022). Defining energy-dense, nutrient-poor food and drinks and estimating the amount of discretionary energy. *Nutrients* 14: https://doi.org/10.3390/nu14071477.

14 Scottish Government (2021). The Scottish health survey 2021: a national statistics publication of Scotland. https://www.gov.scot/binaries/content/documents/govscot/publications/statistics/2018/09/scottish-health-survey-2017-volume-1-main-report/documents/scottish-health-survey-2017-main-report/scottish-health-survey-2017-main-report/govscot%3Adocument/00540654 (accessed 29 March 2024).

15 Malik, V.S. and Hu, F.B. (2022). The role of sugar-sweetened beverages in the global epidemics of obesity and chronic diseases. *Nat. Rev. Endocrinol.* 18: 205–218. https://doi.org/10.1038/s41574-021-00627-6.

16 Keller, A. and Bucher Della Torre, S. (2015). Sugar-sweetened beverages and obesity among children and adolescents: a review of systematic literature reviews. *Child. Obes.* 11: 338–346. https://doi.org/10.1089/chi.2014.0117.

17 von Philipsborn, P., Stratil, J.M., Burns, J. et al. (2019). Environmental interventions to reduce the consumption of sugar-sweetened beverages and their effects on health. *Cochrane Database Syst. Rev.* https://doi.org/10.1002/14651858.CD012292.pub2.

18 WHO (2023). Use of non-sugar sweeteners. https://www.who.int/publications/i/item/9789240046429 (accessed 29 March 2024).

19 NHS Health Scotland (2018). Setting the table. 30341-setting-the-table.pdf (careinspectorate.com) (accessed 29 March 2024).

20 Styne, D.M., Arslanian, S.A., Connor, E.L. et al. (2017). Pediatric obesity-assessment, treatment, and prevention: an endocrine society clinical practice guideline. *J. Clin. Endocrinol. Metab.* 102: 709–757. https://doi.org/10.1210/jc.2016-2573.

21 Dietz, W.H. and Gortmaker, S.L. (1985). Do we fatten our children at the television set? Obesity and television viewing in children and adolescents. *Pediatrics* 75: 807 LP–812 LP. http://pediatrics.aappublications.org/content/75/5/807.abstract.

22 Avery, A., Anderson, C., and McCullough, F. (2017). Associations between children's diet quality and watching television during meal or snack consumption: a systematic review. *Matern. Child. Nutr.* 13: e12428. https://doi.org/10.1111/mcn.12428.

23 Wiecha, J.L., Peterson, K.E., Ludwig, D.S. et al. (2006). When children eat what they watch: impact of television viewing on dietary intake in youth. *Arch. Pediatr. Adolesc. Med.* 160: 436–442. https://doi.org/10.1001/archpedi.160.4.436.

24 Hetherington, M.M., Blundell-Birtill, P., Caton, S.J. et al. (2018). Understanding the science of portion control and the art of downsizing. *Proc. Nutr. Soc.* 77: 347–355. https://doi.org/10.1017/S0029665118000435.

25 Benton, D. (2015). Portion size: what we know and what we need to know. *Crit. Rev. Food Sci. Nutr.* 55: 988–1004. https://doi.org/10.1080/10408398.2012.679980.

26 Nielsen, S.J. and Popkin, B.M. (2004). Changes in beverage intake between 1977 and 2001. *Am. J. Prev. Med.* 27: 205–210. https://doi.org/10.1016/j.amepre.2004.05.005.

27 Hill, J.O. and Peters, J.C. (1998). Environmental contributions to the obesity epidemic. *Science (80-)* 280: 1371–1374. https://doi.org/10.1126/science.280.5368.1371.

28 Wansink, B. and van Ittersum, K. (2006). The visual illusions of food: why plates, bowls, and spoons can bias consumption volume. *FASEB J.* 20: A618–A618. https://doi.org/10.1096/fasebj.20.4.A618-c.

29 Fisher, J.O. and Kral, T.V.E. (2008). Super-size me: portion size effects on young children's eating. *Physiol. Behav.* 94: 39–47. https://doi.org/10.1016/j.physbeh.2007.11.015.

30 Fisher, J.O., Liu, Y., Birch, L.L. et al. (2007). Effects of portion size and energy density on young children's intake at a meal. *Am. J. Clin. Nutr.* 86: 174–179. https://doi.org/10.1093/ajcn/86.1.174.

31 Butland, B., Jebb, S., Kopelman, P. et al. (2007). Tackling obesities: future choices – project report. *Foresight* 162: https://doi.org/10.1002/hep.20263.

32 British Psychology Society (2019). Psychological perspectives on obesity: addressing policy, practice and research priorities. http://doi.org/10.53841/bpsrep.2019.rep130.

33 Pucci, A. and Batterham, R.L. (2020). Endocrinology of the gut and the regulation of body weight and metabolism. In: *Endotext* (ed. K.R. Feingold, B. Anawalt, M.R. Blackman, et al.). South Dartmouth, MA: Endotext.org http://www.ncbi.nlm.nih.gov/pubmed/32352695.

34 American Psychiatric Association (2013). *Diagnostic and Statistical Manual of Mental Disorders: DSM-5TM*, 5e. Arlington, VA: American Psychiatric Publishing, Inc. https://doi.org/10.1176/appi.books.9780890425596.

35 Jebeile, H., Gow, M.L., Baur, L.A. et al. (2019). Treatment of obesity, with a dietary component, and eating disorder risk in children and adolescents: a systematic review with meta-analysis. *Obes. Rev.* 1287–1298. https://doi.org/10.1111/obr.12866.

8 Measuring and Monitoring in Practice

Laura Stewart

'If we think about all the different dimensions there, there is something there about health and well-being part of that and weight and BMI being one part of that as well. So I do think there needs to be more than that. I don't think it can just be down to BMI'. [1]

Introduction

This chapter will explore a range of measurements which could and should be used when assessing and monitoring clinical progress and/or evaluating a childhood weight management service [2]. There are a number of measurements that are discussed, including BMI, psychosocial, medical and person-centred outcomes.

Before using any of the measurements, consideration should be given to whether they are being used for:

- Screening, e.g. for sleep apnoea or eating disorders
- Monitoring clinical progress
- Monitoring service outcomes
- Programme evaluation.

Deciding this will inform which are the most appropriate measurements to use in any particular situation. Other considerations are:

- is the measurement tool age appropriate?
- is the tool the right one to use with a CYP from a particular social or ethnic background?

Child and Adolescent Obesity: A Practical Approach to Clinical Weight Management,
First Edition. Edited by Laura Stewart.
© 2024 John Wiley & Sons Ltd. Published 2024 by John Wiley & Sons Ltd.

For a questionnaire, reflect on the level of literacy that is required for its use. Practically consider the time commitment of the HCP to use the tool, for example the time taken to measure height and weight or to go through a questionnaire with a CYP. Then, if required, take account of the time taken to assess this data, for example calculating and plotting BMI, scoring a questionnaire tool, and having the required clinical reasoning to interpret the result.

The use of BMI, and indeed of taking weight measurements, can sometimes be considered controversial and intrusive. The first section of this chapter will give a brief history of the use of BMI first in adults and then in childhood.

Body Mass Index

BMI is used across the world in epidemiology and clinical practice in childhood obesity diagnosis [3–6]. BMI, whether in adults or children, is calculated using the equation: weight in kilograms divided by height in metres squared.

$$BMI = Wt(kg) \div Ht(m)^2 \text{ or } \left\{ Wt(kg) \div Ht(m) \right\} \div Ht(m)$$

In adults, the number can then be directly related to a weight category (see below), while in children it needs to be plotted on a male/female BMI centile chart [5, 6]. The use of CYP's BMI centile charts has been explored in Chapter 1 and is discussed in further detail in this chapter.

When considering the use of BMI in weight management, the crucial point to understand is that it is used as an everyday, handy (albeit crude) indicator of excess body adiposity (body fat) [7–9]. This is a point that everyone working in weight management requires to thoroughly understand to enable them to interpret and explain BMI in childhood. In a health context, it is not an individual's weight per se, but the level of excess body adiposity, in particular where the excess accumulation is stored around the body, that leads to increased risks of certain health conditions and mortality [8, 9]. These co-morbidities of excess adiposity are well document throughout this book, particularly in Chapter 1. In short these include:

- Type 2 diabetes
- Cardiovascular disease
- Hypertension
- Particular cancers [10, 11].

The Use of BMI in Adults

It is worthwhile considering first the history of use of BMI with adults. There have been many attempts to categorise adult weight as ideal or desirable and/or as a risk factor for poor health or even mortality. Interest in life expectancy and weight became a consideration for life insurance companies when they started to perceive a relationship between body weight and CVD. 'Desirable' weights by frame size of small, medium and large, based on the data from the Metropolitan Life Insurance Company, were frequently used by HCP through the 1960s–1980s [9]. Prof. John Garrow (1981) was a leading exponent for the use of Wt (kg)/Ht² (m²), otherwise known as the Quetelet Index, as first described by the mathematician Dr Adolphe Quetelet in the 1800s that we now refer to as BMI.

BMI helped to move away from the use of small, medium and large frames, with a BMI of 20–25 roughly equivalent to the desirable weight categories of the Metropolitan Life Insurance Companies, with above a BMI of 25 showing an increasing risk of morbidities and mortalities [8]. The WHO published categories for adult BMI in the 1990s and these became widely accepted and used internationally [9].

- underweight <18.5
- ideal/desirable 18.6–24.9
- pre-obesity (overweight) 25.0–29.9
- obesity class I 30.0–34.9
- obesity class II 35.0–39.9
- obesity class III >40 [12].

While these categories are significant in relation to increased risk of morbidity and mortality in adults, at an individual level BMI does not give a measure of body adiposity or an indication of where in the body excess adiposity is stored [8, 12]. Waist measurements are discussed below.

Visceral Body Adiposity

A clinical definition of obesity is in fact relating the risk of disease, morbidity and mortality of the accumulation of excess body adiposity. There is no doubt that the distribution of adiposity, particularly central adiposity, influences these health risks. The evidence shows that it is not simply a central adiposity distribution but more the accumulation of visceral adiposity which is significant in the increased risks of disease [13, 14]. Visceral adiposity is a type of adiposity that is found within the abdominal cavity around visceral organs including the liver, pancreas and intestines. There is no doubt that visceral adiposity accumulation is an important factor in the development of metabolic disease complications, it is indicated as an increased risk and development of type 2 diabetes and CVD. In adults, waist measurement, waist:hip ratio or waist:height ratio is often cited as a more important indicator of potential health risk than BMI. For adults with a BMI below 35 the health risk from central adiposity can be estimated using a waist:height ratio. The NICE updated guidelines stated that in adults, a waist:height ratio 0.5–0.59 indicating increased health risks, while a waist:height ratio of 0.6 and above would indicate further increased health risks [5].

Variation of Adiposity in Childhood

To have an understanding of the BMI centile curves, it is worthwhile very briefly considering the natural variation during childhood of body adiposity, including the differences seen between boys and girls. Humans are born with a small store of adiposity. The early period after birth sees a steady rise of body adiposity and BMI. That then drops during the pre-school toddler years [15] and then starts to increase again until adulthood – the start of this second increase is called adiposity rebound [6]. There is evidence to suggest that an early age of adiposity rebound is associated with an increased risk of later obesity in childhood [16–18]. For females the body naturally stores more body fat than males. This in particular becomes more noticeable for girls during puberty, while during this time boys have a more rapid growth of fat-free mass [15].

The Use of BMI in Children and Young People

BMI is widely used in childhood obesity for clinical diagnosis, service level triaging and public health population monitoring [3, 5, 6]. What still differs across the globe are the BMI cut-off points for defining overweight, obesity and severe obesity. It should be noted that BMI tends not to be used in children under two years of age, mainly due to the difficulty of obtaining an accurate length measurement.

BMI in childhood is calculated using the same equation as for adults. Up until the age of 18 years, the BMI should then be plotted on male/female centile charts for the correct population norms. It is recommended that childhood BMI is best expressed as SD scores (also known as z-scores). While this is correct for research and service evaluation, it would be a complicated process to explain and discuss SD or z-score directly with CYP and their parents. Therefore, in a clinical situation discussing changes in weight, height and BMI with a family is more appropriate.

As in adulthood, any definition of childhood overweight and obesity needs to be able to define not only body fatness but also the clinical relevance of this body fat, i.e. at what level of BMI is there a significant increase in the adverse health risks and consequences of childhood obesity [19]. The specificity and sensitivity of BMI as a tool for diagnosing and classifying some childhood obesity has been discussed in Chapter 1.

In the US, the Center for Disease Control (CDC) produces the BMI centile charts for the US population (*BMI Calculator Child and Teen | Healthy Weight|CDC*). While the UK uses its own BMI centile charts, which incorporates two population norms – the WHO (2009) international data for ages 2–3.9 years old and the UK 1990 data from age 4 years upwards (*Growth charts (rcpch.ac.uk)*).

US BMI Charts

The cut-off points of the 95th centile for obesity, with the 85th centile for overweight, was first used on the USA National Health and Nutrition Examination Surveys (NHANES) charts [6]. Children with a BMI on or over the 95th centile had a higher risk of persistence of obesity in adulthood and of obesity-related diseases [20, 21]. Current US cut-off points for diagnosis and monitoring are outlined in Table 8.1.

UK BMI Charts

Published in the mid-1990s, the UK BMI centile charts were developed by Cole and colleagues, using UK data from 11 studies. These BMI centile charts had nine centile lines, each two thirds of a standard deviation (SD) or z-score apart [22]. For this reason, the UK BMI charts displayed the

Table 8.1 Clinical diagnostic criteria for overweight and obesity in CYP (aged <20 years) in the US [6].

Weight category	US BMI centile range
Underweight	<5th centile
Healthy weight	5th centile to <85th centile
Overweight	85th centile to <95th centile
Obesity	≥95th centile
Severe obesity	≥120% of the 95th centile or ≥ 35 kg/m²
Severe obesity is further defined as:	
Class 2 obesity	BMI ≥120% to <140% of the 95th centile or BMI ≥35 to <40 kg/m²
Class 3 obesity	BMI ≥140% of the 95th centile or BMI ≥40 kg/m²

Source: *Defining Child BMI Categories | Overweight and Obesity | CDC*).

Table 8.2 Clinical diagnostic criteria for overweight and obesity in CYP (aged ≤20 years) in the UK.

Clinical terminology	BMI centiles[a]	SDS or z-score[a]
Overweight	≥91st centile	≥+1.33 SD
Obesity	≥98th centile	≥+2 SD
Severe obesity	≥99.6th centile	≥+2.67 SD
Extreme obesity		+3.33 SD

[a] defined relative to the WHO/UK 1990 reference chart for age and sex.

91st, 98th and 99.6th centile line but not the 85th and 95th centile lines. The Scottish Intercollegiate Guideline Network (SIGN) group in 2003 developed the first UK childhood obesity guidelines and took the pragmatic approach of recommending 91st centile for overweight and 98th centile for obesity in clinical practice while retaining 95th centile for defining obesity and 85th centile for overweight in epidemiological studies [23]. This convention remains in practice in the UK today [3, 5]. The current UK BMI charts now use WHO/UK 1990 data and also show SD lines at 3 SD, 3.33 SD, 3.66 SD and 4 SD (*Body mass index (BMI) chart|RCPCH*). Table 8.2 shows the UK BMI centiles and SD cut-off points for diagnosis and monitoring.

International BMI Charts

In a move to enable monitoring of international prevalence and trends, in 2000 the International Obesity Task Force (IOTF) published their own charts [24]. The IOTF charts are based on cross-sectional growth studies' data combined from the UK, Brazil, Hong Kong, US, the Netherlands and Singapore. For each national BMI dataset data was extrapolated back at the adult definitions of a BMI 25 for overweight (based on adult BMI of 25 at age 18) and a BMI 30 for obesity (based on adult BMI of 30 at age 18). The curves produced with the data were then 'smoothed out' to create two centile lines for the childhood overweight and obesity cut-off points. The IOTF cuts offs sit around the 99th centile for obesity and the 91st centile for overweight when compared to the UK 1990 data [24].

To date there remains no international consensus on the population data, BMI charts and cut-off points to use. In practice, the most important aspect is to understand the accepted practice in your own country, organisation and/or international zone.

Changes in BMI

The most recent Cochrane systematic reviews on childhood weight management treatments gave an idea of BMI changes that can be expected

Table 8.3 Case study example of a 10-year-old girl and treatment effect.

Appt. (Age)	Weight (kg)	Height (m)	Weight change	BMI centile[a]	BMI	BMI SDS
10	50	1.3	–	> 99.6th	29.6	3.14
10½	50.5	1.325	+0.5 kg	> 99.6th	28.8	2.95
11	50.5	1.36	0 kg	< 99.6th	27.3	2.63
		Change +0.06	Change +0.5 kg		Change −2.3	Change of −0.51

[a] WHO/UK1990 Girls BMU chart 2–20 years.
Source: Reproduced with permission from Gahagan and Stewart [7], Wiley-Blackwell

from management programmes. A series of Cochrane systematic reviews have looked at different age ranges:

- <6 years of change a change in BMI SD of −0.3 [25]
- 6–11 years of age a change in BMI SD of −0.04 [26]
- 12–17 years of age a change in BMI of −0.13 [27].

While these figures give an idea of the change in weight and BMI that can be accomplished via a CYP's weight management programme, the systematic reviews still found a concern with the quality of the published research.

Table 8.3 demonstrates that a BMI SD (z-score) change of −0.51 could be seen over the space of 12 months, actually with a small weight increase of 0.5 kg. This decrease in the BMI and BMI SD is actually due to the increases in height and to the nature of the BMI centile curves. Thus, in practice for the majority of CYP, weight maintenance will be an acceptable target. For CYP in the extreme BMI range, particularly with bio-psycho-social complications, consideration of weight loss required needs to be given by the HCP and discussed with the CYP and their parents.

As previously highlighted, in clinical practice, when discussing weight-related interventions with CYP and their parents, outcomes should be measured by weight. In terms of service reviews, evaluations or audits then the indicator to use should be change in BMI SD.

Waist Measurements

McCarthy et al. published data on waist circumference centiles for British children [28]. These centiles were based on cross-sectional data collected in the late 1980s from 3585 males and 4770 females in the UK across a variety of geographical and socio-economic settings. Smoothed centile curves were produced for boys and girls at age intervals. Data was published for 5–16.9 year olds. These waist circumference centiles were for a time on the reverse side of UK BMI centile charts for use in routine clinical practice in the UK.

Waist-to-Height Ratios

There is now a significant move towards using waist:height ratios in CYP as a useful predictor of health risk from visceral fat, with studies showing that it is a valuable index for identifying children at risk of cardiovascular diseases [5]. It can also be useful in monitoring progress through a programme.

In CYP aged 5 years and older, the interpretation of the ratio is similar to that of adults with a:

- waist:height ratio 0.4–0.49, indicating no increased health risks
- waist:height ratio 0.5–0.59, indicating increased health risks
- waist:height ratio of 0.6 and above indicating further increased health risks [5].

Taking Measurements

To be able to calculate BMI and waist:height ratio, measurements need to be taken at regular intervals during a weight management programme. Taking any anthropometric measurements in young people has challenges, particularly with younger children. For anyone working in the field of weight management, the HCP needs to be both confident and competent when taking these measurements. This section gives a brief description of suggested methods to use to ensure consistent and accurate measurements of weight, height, length and waist are taken.

At all times it is important to help the CYP feel comfortable and avoid feeling unsettled by measurements being taken. Therefore, it is vital that the language used is non-judgemental and non-stigmatising, see Chapters 2 and 5.

The equipment used should be fit for purpose. This would include scales that can weigh to necessary weights for the client group, a stadiometer with a fixed head T-plate and a tape measure that is sufficiently long. In the UK, it is recommended that level 3 scales are used, and these should be calibrated annually.

Weight

All CYP should be weighed in as light clothing as possible with outer clothing and heavy clothes such as jumpers and shoes removed. For younger children wearing nappies, these should be removed if possible.

The CYP should be asked to stand in the centre of the scales and be as steady as possible. For some younger children, it may be difficult for them to stand steady on the scales alone and/or it may frighten them. A weight with the parent/carer holding the young child can be taken and then the parent/carer's weight taken and subtracted. It should be noted however that in practice the parent/carer is often very reluctant to have their own weight taken.

Height

Whether taking a length or a height, the CYP's head should be in what is known as the 'Frankfurt Plane'. The Frankfurt Plane requires the eyes to be parallel to the head board/T-bar, the CYP's neck should not be flexed or extended.

For young children under 2 years of age, a length and not a height should be measured. This means that the young child is lying down on a rollameter or a kiddiemeter. Ideally there should be two professionals taking the measurement; however, in practice a parent could help with the measurement. For any length or height measurements, all accessories should be removed from the hair, e.g. a hair bow or scrunchie. For the length, the child's heels and feet should press against the board at the foot with their head in the Frankfurt plane position against the head board. The knees are *gently* pushed down to enable the legs to fully extend. Read and record to the nearest half a centimetre.

For CYP above 2 years, a standing height is required. The young person should be asked to stand as tall as possible, facing outwards with their body touching the stadiometer. They should be facing forward and looking straight ahead. Many stadiometers have feet marks and this helps with the correct direction of facing and position. When the head is in the Frankfurt plane position, the T headboard should be brought down until it sits on the top of the CYP's head. The HCP can use their hands on the CYP's head to ensure that it is sitting in the correct Frankfurt plane position. Read and record to the nearest millimetre [23].

Waist

This is the most challenging measurement to take in a clinical weight management setting. It is exceedingly important to make the CYP feel comfortable and for this many HCPs ask the CYP to pass the measuring tape around their own waist.

The CYP will need to raise their top slightly to allow the tape to be passed around and the correct position to be identified. There are a number of ways described to find the correct position of the waist. In practice taking the waist of CYP with excess weight using the midway point between the lowest rib and the iliac crest is a successful method. The CYP can be asked to bend to one side to pinpoint this particular point. Read and record in millimetres and some recommend that the measurement is repeated three times and then the average used.

Psycho-socio Measurements

While taking anthropometric measurements is important for monitoring clinical progress, reporting on the efficacy of a programme and informing service commissioners, they are not the only measurement that can or should be used. Previous chapters have discussed the well-recognised association between living with obesity and mental well-being. There are vast array of measurement tools that could be used to assess and monitor mental well-being. It is worth considering which measurements are most important for the service and client group to be collected and importantly that can be incorporated into routine in a clinical setting.

The WHO describes mental health as '*a state of mental well-being that enables people to cope with the stresses of life, realize their abilities, learn well and work well, and contribute to their community. It is an integral component of health and well-being that underpins our individual and collective abilities to make decisions, build relationships and shape the world we live in.*' (www.who.int/features/factfiles/mental_health/en/2023)

Many of these tools are frequently seen within research studies and less so in day-to-day clinical practice – so their utilisation and interpretation require careful consideration by a weight management team. Possible tools can be grouped into reporting on anxiety, depression, quality of life (QoL), screening for eating disorder behaviours, and quantifying social outcomes such as school attendance. The list in Table 8.4 is not exhaustive, but gives examples of such tools. Some of these tools can be administered by any HCP in the team, while others require the specialist clinical reasoning of a psychologist for appropriate interpretation of the results. This highlights the importance of multi-disciplinary team working or at a minimum access to a psychologist for support.

Table 8.4 Examples of psycho-socio measurement tools.

Measuring	Tool
Anxiety	Generalised Anxiety Disorder – 7 (GAD-7), <u>Generalised</u> *anxiety disorder questionnaire* | *Diagnosis* | *Generalised anxiety disorder* | *CKS* | *NICE*
Depression	Children's Depression Inventory (CDI) has two forms. `https://www.pearsonclinical.co.uk/store/ukassessments/en/Store/Professional-Assessments/Personality-%26-Biopsychosocial/Brief/Children%27s-Depression-Inventory-2/p/P100009082.html`
Anxiety and depression	Revised Childrens Anxiety and Depression Scale (RCADS) `https://www.corc.uk.net/outcome-experience-measures/revised-childrens-anxiety-and-depression-scale rcads/`
Anxiety and depression	Strengths and Difficulties Questionnaire (SDQ) `https://www.mentallyhealthyschools.org.uk/media/2041/sdq-uk-english-single-side.pdf`
Quality of life	The Impact of Weight on Quality of Life – Kids (IWQOL-Kids) `https://www.qualityoflifeconsulting.com/iwqol-kids.html`
Quality of life	Pediatric Quality of Life Inventory (PedsQL) `https://www.pedsql.org/about_pedsql.html`
School attendance	Self-reported – based on asking 'How many times were you unable to attend school in the past 12 months?'
Self-esteem	Harter's Perceived Competence Scale (1982) `https://www.jstor.org/stable/1129640?origin=crossref`
Dietary behaviours	The Child Eating Behaviour Questionnaire (CEBQ) *Eating behaviour questionnaires* | *Institute of Epidemiology & Health Care – UCL – University College London*
Dietary behaviours	Dutch eating behaviour questionnaire (DEBQ) `https://onlinelibrary.wiley.com/doi/10.1002/1098-108X%2819860 2%295%3A2%3C295%3A%3AAID-EAT2260050209%3E3.0.CO%3B2-T`

Considerations need to be given to the age of the CYP, the culture of the family and to the literacy level of both the CYP and their parents, as well as the time available in the clinic arena to use the tools and the purpose of utilising them. Some of these tools may have been designed for use with older adolescents or indeed adults. Many of the possible tools that could be used will require a license. Any user needs to clarify the copyright status and licensing position before use.

Measuring and Monitoring Lifestyle Behaviour Change

Measuring actual changes in lifestyle behaviour such as diet and physical activity as a routine part of everyday clinical practice is not as easy as might be expected. First, it is important to consider the validity of the chosen tool in actually measuring changes and outcomes being reviewed. Some programmes use simple questions such as time spent in physical activity at the start and completion of the programme. Questionnaires such as the Physical Activity Questionnaire for Older Children (PAQ-C) and the Physical Activity Questionnaire for Adolescents (PAQ-A) are available to be utilised [29]. For dietary changes, food frequency type questions can be used to monitor food intake. An example used by some services would be to ask a few pertinent questions concentrating on particular foods, e.g. sugary drinks, food high in fat and sugar, portions of fruits and vegetables taken per day.

Monitoring Metabolic Complications of Excess Weight in Childhood

In some clinical settings, assessing and then monitoring metabolic complications of obesity will be relevant. In reality, taking these measurements will more than likely only be seen in large teaching hospitals or within a specialist multi-disciplinary childhood weight management team. Viner and Nicholls gave a useful summary of possible clinical investigations for childhood obesity at initial assessment as:

- Baseline bloods
- Fasting glucose
- Fasting insulin
- Fasting lipids (total and HDL cholesterol, triglycerides)
- Liver function (bilirubin and ALT)
- Thyroid function (T4, TSH)
- Full blood count
- Urea and electrolytes
- Blood pressure using an adequate large cuff, comparison to BP centiles for age and sex [30].

Onward referral to specialist teams such as to paediatric endocrinologist or geneticist should be considered, such as for DNA screening for monogenetic forms of obesity, sleep study for obstructive sleep apnoea if there are significant symptoms (snoring, difficult to wake, nightmares, daytime somnolence), and cortisol measurements.

Evaluation of Weight Management Programmes

To ensure the delivery of an appropriate and quality weight management service evaluation is essential. Data collection systems required to be in place including initial assessment and ongoing monitoring [31], not only for clinical feedback but for service-level data interrogation.

While much space has been taken in this chapter discussing clinical outcome measures, equal importance should be given to qualitative measures. Qualitative evaluation and 'patient stories' are a powerful tool for demonstrating the day-to-day outcomes which are most relevant to the CYP and their families [32]. This can be achieved by exploring patient reported experience (PREM's) and patient reported outcome measures (PROMS). On a personal level, for the CYP and/or their parents, clothes size, types or style of clothes or being able to undertake daily functions similar to their peers may be more important outcomes than the number on the scales or a blood pressure reading.

An example of a patient story is that of Daisy, a 10-year-old at referral (Daisy's journey is returned to as a case study in Chapter 11). At initial assessment, it was noted that she was shy with low self-esteem and confidence, had a high level of screen time with little time spent doing physical activity, her parents commented that she had very few friends at school.

On working through a weight management programme for six months, her weight had remained stable with the BMI centile decreasing from 29.6 to 28.8. At the six-month session, Daisy reported that she felt more confident at school and she now had a small friendship group at school. Daisy had reduced her screen time and now has physically activity for at least 30 minutes 5 days each week, much of this time with her friends from school.

WHAT DOES THIS MEAN FOR PRACTICE?

There is widespread international support for the use of BMI to clinically diagnose obesity in children. Despite its well-documented limitations, it is the most practical measure of defining excess body fat in children, provided values are interpreted using relative national child growth references in taking into account age and sex. Waist:height ratio is now recognised as relevant in CYP weight management as a metabolic health risk tool.

HCPs and teams should consider which (if any) psychosocial tools and lifestyle behaviour measurement tools are convenient for them to use in everyday, routine practice, and will give relevant information for the targeted age group. PREMS and PROMS can be useful to use in a routine or ad hoc manner to give qualitative data and add 'real life' colouring to service evaluation.

References

1 Stewart L. (2021). Personal communication: practitioner.
2 Public Health England (2018). Evaluation of weight management, physical activity and dietary interventions: an introductory guide. SEF_weight_management_interventions.pdf (publishing.service.gov.uk) (accessed 29 March 2024).
3 SACN, RCPCH (2012). Position statement: consideration of issues around the use of BMI centile thresholds for defining underweight, overweight and obesity in children aged 2–18 years in the UK. SACN Statement defining child underweight, overweight and obesity – GOV.UK (www.gov.uk) (accessed 29 March 2024).
4 Scottish Intercollegiate Guideline Network (SIGN) (2010). Management of obesity: a national clinical guideline SIGN 115. Edinburgh.
5 NICE (2023). Overview | Obesity: identification, assessment and management | Guidance | NICE (accessed 29 March 2024).
6 Hampl SE, Hassink SG, Skinner AC, et al. Clinical practice guideline for the evaluation and treatment of children and adolescents with obesity. *Pediatrics* 2023;151:e2022060640. https://doi.org/10.1542/peds.2022-060640
7 Gahagan, A. and Stewart, L. (2018). Diagnostic criteria and assessment of obesity in children. In: *Advanced Nutrition and Dietetics in Obesity* (ed. C. Hankey and K. Whelan), 31–37. Wiley-Blackwell.
8 Garrow, J.S. (1981). *Treat Obesity Seriously: A Clinical Manual.* Churchill Livingstone https://books.google.co.uk/books?id=dgRsAAAAMAAJ.
9 Nuttall FQ. Body mass index: obesity, BMI, and health: a critical review. *Nutr. Today* 2015;50:117–28. https://doi.org/10.1097/NT.0000000000000092
10 Reilly JJ, Methven E, Mcdowell ZC, et al. Health consequences of obesity Health consequences of obesity. *JAMA* 2003;:748–52. https://doi.org/10.1136/adc.88.9.748
11 Han JC, Lawlor DA, Kimm SYS. Childhood obesity – 2010: progress and challenges determinants and risk factors for childhood obesity. 2010;375:1737–48. https://doi.org/10.1016/S0140-6736(10)60171-7. Childhood
12 WHO (2000). Obesity: Preventing and Managing the Global Epidemic. Report of a WHO Consultation, Switzerland.
13 Goran, M.I. and Gower, B.A. (1999). Relation between visceral fat and disease risk in children and adolescents. *Am. J. Clin. Nutr.* 70: 149S–156S.

14 Goran, M.I., Bergmen, R.N., and Gower, B.A. (2001). Influence of total vs. visceral fat on insulin action and secretion in African American and white children. *Obes. Res.* 9: 423–431.

15 Wright, C.M. (2015). Defining and measuring childhood obesity. In: *Early Years Nutrition and Healthy Weight* (ed. L. Stewart and J. Thompson), 30–39. Wiley.

16 Dorosty AR, Emmett PM, Cowin SIS, et al. Factors associated with early adiposity rebound. *Pediatrics* 2000;105:1115 LP–1118 LP. https://doi.org/10.1542/peds.105.5.1115

17 Patois E, Guilloud-Bataille M, Rolland-Cachera MF, et al. Adiposity rebound in children: a simple indicator for predicting obesity. *Am. J. Clin. Nutr.* 1984;39:129–35. https://doi.org/10.1093/ajcn/39.1.129

18 Reilly JJ, Armstrong J, Dorosty AR, et al. Early life risk factors for obesity in childhood: cohort study. *BMJ* 2005;330:1357. https://doi.org/10.1136/bmj.38470.670903.E0

19 Maynard LM, Wisemandle W, Roche AF, et al. Childhood body composition in relation to body mass index. *Pediatrics* 2001;107:344 LP–350 LP. https://doi.org/10.1542/peds.107.2.344

20 Barlow SE. Expert Committee recommendations regarding the prevention, assessment, and treatment of child and adolescent overweight and obesity: summary report. *Pediatrics* 2007;120:S164–92. https://doi.org/10.1542/peds.2007-2329c

21 Dietz WH, Robinson TN. Use of the body mass index (BMI) as a measure of overweight in children and adolescents. *J. Pediatr.* 1998;132:191–3. https://doi.org/10.1016/S0022-3476(98)70426-3

22 Tj, C., Jv, F., and Ma, P. (1995). Body mass index reference curves for the. *Arch. Dis. Child.* 73: 25–29.

23 Scottish Intercollegiate Guideline Network (SIGN) (2003). Management of obesity in children and young people. Edinburgh. Our guidelines (sign.ac.uk) (Archived Feb 2020).

24 Cole TJ, Bellizzi MC, Flegal KM, et al. Establishing a standard definition for child overweight and obesity worldwide: international survey. *BMJ Clin. Res. Ed.* 2000;320:1–6. https://doi.org/10.1136/bmj.320.7244.1240

25 Colquitt J, Loveman E, O'Malley C, et al. Diet, physical activity and behavioural interventions for the treatment of overweight or obesity in preschool children up to the age of 6 years (review). Cochrane Database Syst. Rev. 2016. https://doi.org/10.1002/14651858.CD012105

26 Mead E, Brown T, Rees K, et al. Diet, physical activity and behavioural interventions for the treatment of overweight or obese adolescents aged 6 to 11 years (review). Cochrane Database Syst. Rev. 2017. https://doi.org/10.1002/14651858.CD012651

27 Al-Khudairy L, Loveman E, Colquitt JL, et al. Diet, physical activity and behavioural interventions for the treatment of overweight or obese adolescents aged 12 to 17 years. Cochrane Database Syst. Rev. 2017. https://doi.org/10.1002/14651858.CD012691

28 McCarthy HD, Jarrett K V, Crawley HF. The development of waist circumference percentiles in British children aged 5.0–16.9 y. *Eur. J. Clin. Nutr.* 2001;55:902–7. https://doi.org/10.1038/sj.ejcn.1601240

29 Kowalski, K.C., Crocker, P.R.E., Donen, R.M. (2004). The Physical Activity Questionnaire for Older Children (PAQ-C) and Adolescents (PAQ-A) Manual. `The_Physical_Activity_Questionnaire_for_Older_Chil.pdf` (accessed 01 March 2024).

30 Viner R, Nicholls D. Managing obesity in secondary care: a personal practice. *Arch. Dis. Child.* 2005;90:385–90. `https://doi.org/10.1136/adc.2004.062224`

31 Public Health England (2018). Standard Evaluation Framework for Weight Management Interventions Standard Evaluation Framework for Weight Management Interventions.

32 Weldring T, Smith SMS. Article commentary: patient-reported outcomes (PROs) and patient-reported outcome measures (PROMs). *Heal. Serv. Insights* 2013;6:HSI.S11093. `https://doi.org/10.4137/hsi.s11093`.

9 Understanding Obesity in Early Life

Julie Lanigan

'Working with families as early as possible to try to establish those healthier habits, healthier routines and also follow them through'. [1]

Introduction

Childhood obesity is a cause for concern and challenge to healthcare services across the world [2]. Obesity is a disease; and the path begins early in life. In 2016, the WHO estimated that more than 41 million children under five have overweight or obesity [3]. Excess weight gain affects children of all ages in countries around the world, including high and low-to-middle income countries. Once gained, excess weight is difficult to lose and obesity soon becomes established. This is a major concern for global public health, as carrying excess weight in childhood has adverse effects on health in the short and long term. In the short term, children with excess weight are at increased risk of diseases including asthma and sleep apnoea [4]. Both of which can have serious health consequences. Having excess wright in childhood affects both physical and mental health. For example, children with excess weight may have reduced self-esteem, are more likely to be bullied than healthy weight children and to suffer obesity associated stigma [5]. Obesity tracks through childhood and often persists into adult life, where it is associated with increased risk of chronic diseases including those affecting the cardiovascular system (hypertension, dyslipidaemia, type II diabetes) and certain cancers [6]. Prevention of obesity is therefore of the utmost importance. The early years are an opportunity for interventions to reduce the risk of overweight and obesity.

Child and Adolescent Obesity: A Practical Approach to Clinical Weight Management, First Edition. Edited by Laura Stewart.
© 2024 John Wiley & Sons Ltd. Published 2024 by John Wiley & Sons Ltd.

Understanding risk factors is key to successful intervention. This chapter summarises the causes of obesity development in early life and considers possible adverse effects on health and potential interventions for risk reduction.

Risk Factors for Obesity in Childhood

A myriad of factors interacts to increase the risk of obesity. Broadly speaking, these can be categorised as genetic or environmental. Environmental risk factors include less healthy diets, low levels of physical activity and high sedentary behaviour. More recently, behavioural factors that influence dietary and physical activity habits have emerged as important in the development of overweight and obesity.

Genetic Risk Factors for Obesity

Genetic factors influence the development of obesity in predisposed individuals [7]. This can be seen where obesity presents in parents and children from the same family. Having at least one parent with obesity increases the likelihood of excess weight in the child, and where both parents are affected, the risk may be up to tenfold of that in children with non-affected parents. In fact, adoption and twin studies suggest that between 40 and 70% of the tendency to obesity is heritable [8]. Genetic studies have identified multiple genes linked to increased risk of obesity. However, only a small proportion of the variation seen in BMI can be explained by genetics [9]. Obesity is mostly polygenic which means that many genes influence risk but individually each gene has small effects. Very few genes have been identified that can individually lead to severe obesity. The most well studied of these are the MC4R and fat mass and obesity-related (FTO) genes [10]. Genetic factors are important, but not all susceptible individuals become overweight. This suggests that environmental factors play a crucial role in the development of obesity.

Environmental Risk Factors for Obesity

In simple terms, overweight and obesity develop when energy intake from dietary sources (foods and beverages) is greater than what is needed for metabolism, activity and growth causing an imbalance. If sustained over a significant period, energy imbalance can lead to weight gain as excess energy is converted to adipose tissue (fat) and stored on the body.

Environmental risk factors for obesity include multiple features of systems that expose individuals to an 'obesogenic' environment, including high availability of energy dense foods and beverages that are easily affordable. Family, socioeconomic, ecological, and biological factors interact to influence risk. All children are at risk but those from poorer backgrounds are worse affected. For example, obesity prevalence in the most socially deprived proportion of the population in England was double that of the least deprived portion according to the most recent report from the National Child Measurement Programme (NCMP). Social determinants of health have a major impact on obesity. For example, disadvantaged families are more likely to have reduced access to green spaces for physical activity [11] and live in proximity to food outlets selling less healthy foods [12]. Less healthy diets, low levels of physical activity and higher times spent sedentary are key environmental risk factors. However, dietary risk factors are suggested to have the greatest impact on excess weight gain [4].

Dietary Risk Factors in Early Life

Nutrition has a central role in the development of overweight or obesity from very early in life. For instance, infant feeding method has been shown to influence weight gain. Breastfeeding, and in particular exclusive breastfeeding for a longer duration, has a moderate protective effect against obesity as reviewed by Victora [13]. Therefore, an important public health message is to breastfeed exclusively for the first six months of life, as recommended by WHO [14]. Not all mothers are able to breastfeed however, and some choose not to do so. For these mothers, infant formula is the only alternative food. Studies have shown that formula-fed infants grow more rapidly during infancy than those breastfed and have an increased risk of obesity in later childhood [15, 16]. It is unclear why this happens, but it is suggested that higher protein in infant formulas may drive more rapid growth [17]. Infant feeding behaviours and parental feeding styles also play a key role in modulation of growth. To reduce the risk of rapid weight gain, responsive feeding, where a mother responds appropriately to her infant's cues as they signal hunger or satiety is best practice. This is particularly relevant to formula-fed infants who are less able to self-regulate their intake compared with breastfed infants [18]. Beyond the first six months of life, when milk is the sole source of nutrition, complementary feeding, when solids are introduced, is a critical period for growth. Feeding practices during this period may increase the risk of excess weight gain.

Complementary Feeding and Risk of Obesity

The complementary feeding (or weaning) period is a transitional time when lifelong dietary habits are established. From about six months, milk alone is unable to meet the nutritional needs of infants who are growing and developing relatively rapidly [19]. During this time, the diet must be expanded to include foods from all the major groups so that the infant can meet their nutritional needs. The aim of complementary feeding is to establish a varied diet that meets all nutritional requirements but is not excessive in energy or specific nutrients.

Studies investigating relationships between complementary feeding and risk of obesity have mostly focussed on the age of infants at introduction of complementary foods. Studies consistently report that early introduction of complementary foods (before four months) is linked to an increased risk of obesity later in childhood as reviewed by Wang [20]. For example, the introduction of complementary foods before four months was associated with a one third increased risk of later obesity compared with introduction after four months (relative risk, 1.33; 95% CI: 1.07–1.64) [20]. Most studies in this review were observational and unable to define causality. Therefore, reverse causality cannot be ruled out, and it is unknown whether larger babies were given complementary foods earlier, as parents and caregivers perceived them to be ready, or if earlier feeding led to larger babies. Consistency of findings, however, suggests complementary foods should be introduced after four months to reduce the risk of later obesity [19]. Timing of introduction of solid foods is important. However, the type and quantity of foods provided play a major role.

Energy intake during complementary feeding must be sufficient to meet needs for growth and development in the rapidly growing infant. Infants and small children have limited stomach capacity. Therefore, a relatively energy dense diet is needed. However, higher intake of energy dense foods during complementary feeding has been linked to rapid weight gain and increased risk of obesity [19]. It is unclear which foods and nutrients contribute most to excess weight gain during complementary feeding. Studies have found no association between fat and carbohydrate intake and excess weight gain. However, higher protein intake is consistently associated with increased risk of childhood obesity, as reviewed [21]. Protein intake increases markedly after the onset of complementary feeding and constitutes 15% of energy compared with 5% during the sole milk feeding period [22].

Behavioural factors during complementary feeding also play an important role in the development of obesity. Healthy growth depends not only on when and what an infant is fed but also on how feeding is done. As with milk feeding, it is important that parents and caregivers practice responsive feeding during the transition from milk to the foods the family eat. An authoritative feeding style (see Chapter 10), where the caregiver responds appropriately to an infant's demandingness is reported to be the most supportive of healthy growth [23].

Baby-led weaning is one approach to complementary feeding that has become popular [24]. The baby-led weaning method encourages self-feeding in infants and has been suggested as protective against the development of obesity. Observational studies suggest that infants fed using the baby-led weaning approach have higher satiety responsiveness [25]. This may offer greater protection against overweight in later childhood compared with those weaned traditionally using spoon feeding [26]. Objective research in this field is limited however and the only two randomised controlled trials (RCTs) are conflicting. For example, an RCT in UK infants found no difference in obesity risk at preschool age in children randomised to baby-led weaning compared with controls following standard advice (difference in BMI z-score at age 2, 0.16; 95% CI: −0.123 to 0.45) [26] while a study in Turkey found that infants traditionally spoon fed had a higher risk of obesity at 1 year of age compared with a baby-led weaning group [27]. Available data are insufficient to inform public health recommendations regarding the method of complementary feeding and risk of obesity and further research is needed to clarify these relationships. Beyond complementary feeding, the preschool diet has also been a focus of research into the development of childhood obesity.

Preschool Diet and Risk of Obesity

Diets of preschool children have changed markedly since the onset of the obesity epidemic. National surveys and studies consistently report that diets of young children do not comply with recommendations [28]. Typically, preschool children's diets are low in fruit, vegetables, and fibre, while high in saturated fat and sugar. Most studies investigating which components of the preschool diet are most strongly related to obesity risk have focused on energy intake. Findings are conflicting with some studies reporting that children with obesity have higher energy intakes than those of healthy weight [29, 30], while others have found the opposite [31, 32]. Most studies investigating energy intake are observational and rely on self-reported intake. Few studies use objective measures to estimate energy expenditure, and most have been conducted in adults. These studies consistently report that adults with obesity underestimate intake [33]. This is also likely to apply to children where estimates of dietary intake rely on parental reports [34].

Evaluating relationships between diet and obesity is complex and interpretation is hampered by heterogeneity of studies that are often not purposefully designed to address such questions and may lack scientific rigour. For example, many studies have small sample sizes and thereby may lack the power needed to detect small but important differences in energy intake that can influence weight gain [35]. Laboratory-based energy balance studies have shown that relatively small excesses in energy intake above requirements, if sustained over time, can lead to energy imbalance and weight gain [35]. Another possible explanation is that lower energy expenditure rather than higher energy intake is the main determinant of obesity. However, studies using objective measures of energy expenditure and metabolisable intake (the gold standard of doubly labelled water) do not support this idea [35].

In summary, available evidence does not support that higher energy intake is associated with increased risk of obesity in young children. However, energy balance is key to achieving and maintaining a healthy weight, and avoiding excessive energy intake in young children is recommended.

Regular growth monitoring is essential in the identification of excessive weight gain in young children. Growth in young children should be evaluated according to appropriate reference data. The WHO multi-centre breastfed growth reference standards are based on data derived from breastfed infants growing under optimal conditions, and these can be used to identify children gaining weight more rapidly and at increased risk of obesity [36].

Studies investigating relationships between macronutrients and risk of obesity in preschool children are limited. Fat, as the most energy dense macronutrient, is a candidate nutrient driving weight gain and has been the focus of research. In a review, Agostoni [37] found no association between the amount or type of fat consumed by preschool children and risk of obesity in later childhood [37]. Carbohydrate is also a major energy source in children's diets and the focus of much research. However, studies have found no associations between carbohydrate intake in preschool and risk of later obesity [38]. As with infants, protein is the macronutrient most strongly associated with obesity risk in preschool children. A meta-analysis of 17 studies found that higher protein intake during preschool was associated with a higher BMI later in childhood (0.28 BMI z-scores, 95% CI: 0.20–0.35) [20]. The effect may be large. In one study of 2000 preschool children, a small increase in protein intake (1%) was associated with a 0.04 unit increase in BMI at the age of 5 [39]. Similarly, a study of 3000 children from the Netherlands found that a 10 g/day increase in protein intake at one year was associated with higher BMI and fat mass in later childhood [40].

The mechanisms underlying associations of higher protein intake with obesity risk are unclear. However, it has been suggested that higher protein diets may promote faster growth through programming effects on insulin-like growth factor-1 (IGF-1) [22]. Evidence is currently limited to only a few observational studies, and further research is needed to confirm this hypothesis.

Studies investigating associations of specific foods and beverages with risk of obesity in preschool children have proved more informative. Evidence suggests high intake of cow's milk promotes growth and excess weight gain. In view of this, it is recommended that cow's milk, given as a main drink, does not exceed 500 ml/day in preschool children [19].

Sugar consumption in preschool children has increased in parallel with the obesity epidemic, prompting research into relationships between foods high in sugar and obesity risk. Sugar-sweetened beverages (SSB) have been a focus of this research. SSB consumption in childhood has a significant impact on obesity and associated metabolic risks, including insulin resistance, type 2 diabetes, hypertension, and metabolic syndrome as reviewed by Calcaterra [41]. Factors influencing SSB consumption in children include socioeconomic status, individual child and parental characteristics and behaviours. Further research is needed before firm conclusions can be made regarding the relationship of SSB with obesity risk in young children. However, in view of the concurrent rise in sugar intake and obesity prevalence, high sugar foods are likely to contribute to obesity risk in this age group and advice to reduce intake is warranted.

Beyond specific foods and nutrients, overall dietary patterns have captured the interest of researchers investigating diets in preschool children and obesity risk.

Dietary Patterns in Preschool Children and Risk of Obesity

Dietary patterns are derived from food intake data using principal component analysis. This method reduces large data sets to fewer variables by combining highly correlated factors. Foods commonly consumed together are combined to form groups and identify dietary patterns that are named according to predominating foods. Dietary patterns emerge early in childhood and become established by the age of 3 years [42]. Once established dietary patterns are stable and track through childhood [43]. This can be a concern as less healthy dietary patterns, characterised by high intake of energy dense foods and low intake of fruits, vegetables and fibre, are associated with obesity in children [44].

Only a few studies have investigated associations between dietary patterns and obesity risk in infants and young children with differing results. One study found that a dietary pattern characterised by later introduction of dairy foods and high use of readily prepared baby foods in infancy was associated with rapid growth between one and three years [45]. Another study in Australia found no association of dietary patterns in toddlers with risk of obesity in later childhood [46]. Findings should be interpreted with caution as dietary patterns provide broad information on diet quality and can only explain a small proportion of the variance in outcomes. More research is needed before firm conclusions can be drawn on the influences of specific dietary patterns on obesity risk in young children.

As discussed earlier, weight gain is the result of an imbalance between energy intake from food and beverages and expenditure. Energy intake depends on the amount and frequency of food consumed which is influenced by portion size and meal and snack occasions. Recent research has investigated associations between portion size, meal frequency and obesity risk in young children.

Portion Size

Children's portions have increased markedly in size over the past three decades in line with the sharp rise in obesity [47]. Although infants and young children can self-regulate energy intake, evidence suggests this can be overridden. Studies have found that children will eat more when given the opportunity. One of the earliest studies investigating this found that providing larger portions to preschool children led to higher food and energy intake [48]. This 'portion size effect' was not seen in younger children. While serving larger portions led to higher intake in 5-year-old children, 3-year-olds did not eat more. This supports that children have an innate ability for appetite regulation in early childhood [48]. However, the study does not tell us whether larger portion sizes increase obesity risk. Syrad investigated associations between meal size and growth in preschool children [49]. Larger meal size between two and five years was associated with more rapid weight gain suggesting portion size could be a risk factor for obesity in young children [49].

In summary, evidence suggests that diet during preschool is important in the development of obesity. Dietary components, patterns and amounts consumed have all been associated with excess weight gain. The strongest evidence for a role of specific nutrients in excess weight gain is for an association of higher protein intake. Larger portion size has been linked to higher intake and faster growth. However, further research is needed to inform appropriate portion sizes for preschool children taking individual variation into account. More information on dietary patterns across the preschool age range is needed to improve understanding of dietary quality and its influence on obesity risk.

Nutrition and diet are key risk factors for obesity and are one component of energy balance. On the other side of the equation, physical activity is also an important consideration when assessing obesity risk (see also Chapter 6).

Physical Activity and Sedentary Behaviours in Preschool Children

Studies and surveys consistently report that preschool children fall short of recommendations for daily physical activity [50, 51]. For example, in the United Kingdom, only 10% of children aged 2–4 years met recommendations for three hours of physical activity daily in 2011 [52]. This is a concern as low levels of total physical activity are associated with a higher risk of obesity in children, as reviewed by te Velde [53].

Not surprisingly, a low level of total physical activity is associated with more time spent sedentary, another independent risk factor for obesity [54]. Studies suggest preschool children are spending excessive time in sedentary behaviours, as reviewed by Downing [55]. For instance, time spent sedentary, including watching TV and spending time on devices, ranged from 37 to 330 minutes daily in young children [55]. Relationships between screen time in preschool children and obesity risk in later childhood are poorly understood. A study from Canada found that an extra 75 minutes watching TV at preschool age was associated with a 13% increase in BMI in teenagers [56].

Shorter sleep duration in early childhood (<10 hours) has been suggested as a risk factor for obesity, as reviewed by Chen. The mechanisms are unclear, but it has been suggested that this may operate through negative effects of shorter sleep on appetite regulation and energy balance [57]. This is supported by at least one study, which found that shorter sleep duration in preschool children (<10.5 hours) was associated with a higher risk of obesity at seven years (odds ratio: 1.45; 95% CI: 1.10, 1.89) [58]. Further research would help confirm this finding and its relevance to diverse populations.

Developmental Risk Factors

Evidence suggests that developmental factors, operative in early life, programme later obesity. Available evidence is largely observational although a small number of experimental studies support this hypothesis. A systematic review confirmed that maternal and child factors are associated with increased obesity risk [59]. The strongest predictors of later obesity in the child were maternal BMI prior to pregnancy, gestational weight gain, exposure to tobacco during pregnancy, infant size at birth and rate of neonatal weight gain. To a lesser extent, socioeconomic factors, sleep duration, parental feeding styles and complementary feeding practices were implicated. It is important to note that studies investigating associations between risk factors and obesity are subject to confounding factors. For example, mothers of higher SES have been reported as more likely to breastfeed, and higher SES is associated with lower risk of obesity. In other words, factors that make a mother more likely to breastfeed may also be a confounding factor protecting against obesity risk in children.

Nutrition and Growth

Strong evidence supports that rapid growth in infancy increases the risk of later obesity. Breastfed infants grow more slowly than formula-fed infants and are less prone to obesity. The benefits of breastfeeding for obesity prevention are proposed to relate to this slower pattern of growth in breastfed infants which is suggested to programme susceptibility to obesity [60]. This is supported by several systematic reviews that found rapid growth in infancy is strongly associated with increased risk of obesity [15, 16, 61]. Mechanisms are not fully understood but may include effects on endocrine systems regulating appetite, food intake, energy storage and fat deposition [62]. Growth trajectories can be influenced for long-term health benefit and to reduce the risk of excess weight gain, as discussed in the WHO New Framework for Prevention and Management of Obesity [63]. This report highlights the importance of establishing healthy dietary and physical activity behaviours to reduce risk.

Overview

The causes of obesity in early life are complex and no one causal factor has so far been identified. Evidence supports lifestyle factors including diet, physical activity and related behaviours as key targets for interventions. The aim of interventions in this age group is to prevent rather than treat obesity by reducing risk. Available evidence suggests this can best be achieved by optimising nutrition and growth in infancy and instilling healthy lifestyle behaviours (e.g. dietary and physical activity related) that are taken forward into later childhood. Interventions to prevent obesity in early life are discussed briefly in the following sections.

Interventions to Prevent Obesity in Early Life

Interventions with some evidence to show they are effective in prevention of obesity are available worldwide. Systematic reviews and meta-analyses have found that successful interventions address dietary and physical activity behaviours together. The largest effects are seen in children below the age of 6 [64]. Few studies report long-term follow-up. Therefore, evidence for sustainable effects of interventions is largely lacking.

Planet Munch is one intervention that was developed in the United Kingdom and evaluated using a randomised controlled study design.

The Planet Munch Healthy Lifestyle Programme for Preschool Children

Planet Munch (formerly known as TrimTots) is a 24-week multi-component programme for obesity prevention in preschool children with an emphasis on family participation and learning through art and play. This is the only preschool intervention for obesity prevention in the United Kingdom that integrates the NICE recommendations in a single comprehensive programme that has been evaluated in randomised controlled trials and shown to be effective at reducing obesity and risk factors. To assess feasibility, Planet Munch was evaluated in two small-scale RCTs. Trial 1 included children classified as overweight (BMI at or above the 91st centile on the WHO/UK 1990 growth reference) or who were at increased risk of becoming overweight (having one parent with excess weight or had experienced rapid growth in infancy). BMI was significantly lower at the end of the programme in the intervention group compared with waiting list controls (mean difference in BMI z-score: -0.9; 95% CI: -1.4 to -0.4, $P = 0.001$). Importantly, this effect was sustained up to 2 years after completing the intervention. BMI was lower in children after participation in the programme compared with baseline (mean difference in BMI z-score: -0.3, 95% CI: -0.6 to -0.1, $P = 0.007$). In a second trial, Planet Munch was evaluated in the general preschool population and found to be effective at reducing risk of overweight and obesity [65].

Planet Munch has been successfully adapted for delivery in multicultural settings in the United Kingdom and overseas. Research that aims to evaluate feasibility in these settings is underway. A larger-scale cluster randomised controlled trial is planned to evaluate efficacy in the wider UK population.

WHAT **DOES** THIS MEAN FOR PRACTICE?

Childhood obesity is a burgeoning problem that presents considerable health risks for future generations. Public health and individual level interventions with evidence of long-term success are scarce.

Multi-component lifestyle prevention programmes are one strategy that can help reduce the risk of childhood obesity. These should be tailored to meet the needs of families and children within their cultural setting while targeting both diet and physical activity improvements. Interventions are urgently needed across the world to prevent the rise in obesity in our youngest children.

References

1 Stewart, L. (2021). Personal communication: practitioner.
2 NCD Risk Factor Collaboration (NCD-RisC) Worldwide trends in body-mass index, underweight, overweight, and obesity from 1975 to 2016: a pooled analysis of 2416 population-based measurement studies in 128·9 million children, adolescents, and adults. *Lancet* 2017 (390): 2627–2642.
3 World Health Organisation (2018). Obesity and overweight fact sheet. Geneva. https://www.who.int/news-room/fact-sheets/detail/obesity-and-overweight (accessed 29 April 2024).
4 Davies, S.C. (2019). *Time to Solve Childhood Obesity*. Department of Health Social Care https://www.gov.uk/government/organisations/department-of-health-and-social-care (accessed 29 April 2024).
5 Sjoberg, R.L., Nilsson, K.W., and Leppert, J. (2005). Obesity, shame, and depression in school-aged children: a population-based study. *Pediatrics* 116: e389–e392.
6 Cunningham, S.A., Kramer, M.R., and Narayan, K.M.V. (2014). Incidence of childhood obesity in the United States. *N. Engl. J. Med.* 370: 403–411.
7 Sheikh, A.B., Nasrullah, A., Haq, S. et al. (2017). The interplay of genetics and environmental factors in the development of obesity. *Cureus* 9: e1435.
8 Loos, R.J.F. and Yeo, G.S.H. (2022). The genetics of obesity: from discovery to biology. *Nat. Rev. Genet.* 23: 120–133.
9 Elks, C.E., den Hoed, M., Zhao, J.H. et al. (2012). Variability in the heritability of body mass index: a systematic review and meta-regression. *Front. Endocrinol. (Lausanne)* 3: 29. https://doi.org/10.3389/fendo.2012.00029. eCollection.
10 Goodarzi, M.O. (2018). Genetics of obesity: what genetic association studies have taught us about the biology of obesity and its complications. *Lancet Diabet. Endocrinol.* 6: 223–236.
11 Shoari, N., Ezzati, M., Doyle, Y.G. et al. (2021). Nowhere to play: available open and green space in greater London schools. *J. Urban Health* 98: 375–384.
12 Han, J., Schwartz, A.E., and Elbel, B. (2020). Does proximity to fast food cause childhood obesity? Evidence from public housing. *Reg. Sci. Urban Econ.* 84: 103565.
13 Victora, C.G., Bahl, R., Barros, A.J. et al. (2016). Breastfeeding in the 21st century: epidemiology, mechanisms, and lifelong effect. *Lancet* 387: 475–490.
14 WHO (2024). Infant Feeding Recommendation (to be added) WHO Guideline for complementary feeding of infants and young children 6–23 months of age. https://www.who.int/publications/i/item/9789240081864 (accessed 29 April 2024).
15 Baird, J., Fisher, D., Lucas, P. et al. (2005). Being big or growing fast: systematic review of size and growth in infancy and later obesity. *BMJ* 331: 929.
16 Monteiro, P.O. and Victora, C.G. (2005). Rapid growth in infancy and childhood and obesity in later life – a systematic review. *Obes. Rev.* 6: 143–154.

17 Ren, Q., Li, K., Sun, H. et al. (2022). The association of formula protein content and growth in early infancy: a systematic review and meta-analysis. *Nutrients* 11: 2255.

18 Li, R., Magadia, J., Fein, S.B., and Grummer-Strawn, L.M. (2012). Risk of bottle-feeding for rapid weight gain during the first year of life. *Arch. Pediatr. Adolesc. Med.* 166: 431–436.

19 Fewtrell, M., Bronsky, J., Campoy, C. et al. (2017). Complementary feeding: a position paper by the European Society for Paediatric Gastroenterology, Hepatology, and Nutrition (ESPGHAN) Committee on Nutrition. *J. Pediatr. Gastroenterol. Nutr.* 64: 119–132.

20 Wang, J., Wu, Y., Xiong, G. et al. (2016). Introduction of complementary feeding before 4months of age increases the risk of childhood overweight or obesity: a meta-analysis of prospective cohort studies. *Nutr. Res.* 36: 759–770.

21 Lanigan, J. (2018). Prevention of overweight and obesity in early life. *Proc. Nutr. Soc.* 77: 247–256.

22 Lind, M.V., Larnkjaer, A., Molgaard, C. et al. (2017). Dietary protein intake and quality in early life: impact on growth and obesity. *Curr. Opin. Clin. Nutr. Metab. Care* 20: 71–76.

23 Kong, K.L., Anzman-Frasca, S., Burgess, B. et al. (2023). Systematic review of general parenting intervention impacts on child weight as a secondary outcome. *Child. Obes.* 19: 5.

24 Taylor, R.W., Williams, S.M., Fangupo, L.J. et al. (2017). Effect of a baby-led approach to complementary feeding on infant growth and overweight: a randomized clinical trial. *JAMA Pediatr.* 171: 838–846.

25 Brown, A. and Lee, M.D. (2015). Early influences on child satiety-responsiveness: the role of weaning style. *Pediatr. Obes.* 10: 57–66.

26 Townsend, E. and Pitchford, N.J. (2012). Baby knows best? The impact of weaning style on food preferences and body mass index in early childhood in a case-controlled sample. *BMJ Open.* 2: e000298.

27 Dogan, E., Yilmaz, G., Caylan, N. et al. (2018). Baby-led complementary feeding: randomized controlled study. *Pediatr. Int.* 60 (12): 1073–1080.

28 NDNS (2011). *National Diet and Nutrition Survey: Headline Results from Years 1 and 2 (Combined) of the Rolling Programme (2008/2009–2009/10)*. London: HMSO.

29 Anderson, E.L., Tilling, K., Fraser, A. et al. (2013). Estimating trajectories of energy intake through childhood and adolescence using linear-spline multilevel models. *Epidemiology* 24: 507–515.

30 Hebestreit, A., Bornhorst, C., Pala, V. et al. (2014). Dietary energy density in young children across Europe. *Int. J. Obes.* 38 (Suppl 2): S124–S134.

31 Rocandio, A.M., Ansotegui, L., and Arroyo, M. (2001). Comparison of dietary intake among overweight and non-overweight schoolchildren. *Int. J. Obes. Relat. Metab. Disord.* 25: 1651–1655.

32 Niinikoski, H., Viikari, J., Ronnemaa, T. et al. (1997). Regulation of growth of 7- to 36-month-old children by energy and fat intake in the prospective, randomized STRIP baby trial. *Pediatrics* 100: 810–816.

33 Swinburn, B., Sacks, G., and Ravussin, E. (2009). Increased food energy supply is more than sufficient to explain the US epidemic of obesity. *Am. J. Clin. Nutr.* 90: 1453–1456.

34 Foster, E., Hawkins, A., Barton, K.L. et al. (2017). Development of food photographs for use with children aged 18 months to 16 years: comparison against weighed food diaries – The Young Person's Food Atlas (UK). *PLoS One* 12: e0169084.

35 Hill, J.O., Wyatt, H.R., and Peters, J.C. (2012). Energy balance and obesity. *Circulation* 126: 126–132.

36 de Onis, M., Garza, C., Victora, C.G. et al. (2004). The WHO Multicentre Growth Reference Study: planning, study design, and methodology. *Food Nutr. Bull.* 25 (1 Suppl): S15–S26.

37 Agostoni, C. and Caroli, M. (2012). Role of fats in the first two years of life as related to later development of NCDs. *Nutr. Metab. Cardiovasc. Dis.* 22: 775–780.

38 Patro-Gołąb, B., Zalewski, B.M., Kołodziej, M. et al. (2016). Nutritional interventions or exposures in infants and children aged up to 3 years and their effects on subsequent risk of overweight, obesity and body fat: a systematic review of systematic reviews. *Obes. Rev.* 17: 1245–1257.

39 Pimpin, L., Jebb, S., Johnson, L. et al. (2016). Dietary protein intake is associated with body mass index and weight up to 5 y of age in a prospective cohort of twins. *Am. J. Clin. Nutr.* 103: 389–397.

40 Voortman, T., Braun, K.V., Kiefte-de Jong, J.C. et al. (2016). Protein intake in early childhood and body composition at the age of 6 years: The Generation R Study. *Int. J. Obes.* 40: 1018–1025.

41 Calcaterra, V., Cena, H., Comola, V.C.M.A.V.G. et al. (2023). Sugar-sweetened beverages and metabolic risk in children and adolescents with obesity: a narrative review. *Nutrients* 15 (3): 702.

42 North, K. and Emmett, P. (2000). Multivariate analysis of diet among three-year-old children and associations with socio-demographic characteristics. The Avon Longitudinal Study of Pregnancy and Childhood (ALSPAC) Study Team. *Eur. J. Clin. Nutr.* 54: 73–80.

43 Mikkila, V., Rasanen, L., Raitakari, O.T. et al. (2005). Consistent dietary patterns identified from childhood to adulthood: the cardiovascular risk in Young Finns Study. *Br. J. Nutr.* 93: 923–931.

44 Ambrosini, G.L. (2014). Childhood dietary patterns and later obesity: a review of the evidence. *Proc. Nutr. Soc.* 73: 137–146.

45 Betoko, A., Lioret, S., Heude, B. et al. (2017). Influence of infant feeding patterns over the first year of life on growth from birth to 5 years. *Pediatr. Obes.* 12 (Suppl. 1): 94–101.

46 Bell, L.K., Golley, R.K., and Daniels, L. (2013). Dietary patterns of Australian children aged 14 and 24 months, and associations with socio-demographic factors and adiposity. *Eur. J. Clin. Nutr.* 67: 638–645.

47 Small, L., Lane, H., Vaughan, L. et al. (2013). A systematic review of the evidence: the effects of portion size manipulation with children and portion education/training interventions on dietary intake with adults. *Worldviews Evid. Based Nurs.* 10: 69–81.

48 Rolls, B.J., Engell, D., and Birch, L.L. (2000). Serving portion size influences 5-year-old but not 3-year-old children's food intakes. *J. Am. Diet. Assoc.* 100: 232–234.

49 Syrad, H., Llewellyn, C.H., Johnson, L. et al. (2016). Meal size is a critical driver of weight gain in early childhood. *Sci. Rep.* 6: 28368.

50 Reilly, J.J. (2008). Physical activity, sedentary behaviour and energy balance in the preschool child: opportunities for early obesity prevention. *Proc. Nutr. Soc.* 67: 317–325.

51 Goldfield, G.S., Harvey, A., Grattan, K. et al. (2012). Physical activity promotion in the preschool years: a critical period to intervene. *Int. J. Environ. Res. Publ. Health* 9: 1326–1342.

52 Tinner, L., Kipping, R., White, J. et al. (2019). Cross-sectional analysis of physical activity in 2–4-year-olds in England with paediatric quality of life and family expenditure on physical activity. *BMC Publ. Health* 19: 846.

53 te Velde, S.J., Van, N.F., Uijtdewilligen, L. et al. (2012). Energy balance-related behaviours associated with overweight and obesity in preschool children: a systematic review of prospective studies. *Obes. Rev.* 13 (Suppl. 1): 56–74.

54 De Craemer M, De Decker E, de Bourdeaudhuij I et al. Correlates of energy balance-related behaviours in preschool children: a systematic review. Obes. Rev. (2012) 13, Suppl. 1, 13–28.

55 Downing, K.L., Hnatiuk, J., and Hesketh, K.D. (2015). Prevalence of sedentary behavior in children under 2 years: a systematic review. *Prev. Med.* 78: 105–114.

56 Simonato, I., Janosz, M., Archambault, I., and Pagani, L.S. (2018). Prospective associations between toddler televiewing and subsequent lifestyle habits in adolescence. *Prev. Med.* 7 (110): 24–30.

57 Chen, X., Beydoun, M.A., and Wang, Y. (2008). Is sleep duration associated with childhood obesity? A systematic review and meta-analysis. *Obesity* 16: 265–274.

58 Reilly, J.J., Armstrong, J., Dorosty, A.R. et al. (2005). Early life risk factors for obesity in childhood: cohort study. *BMJ* 330: 1357.

59 Woo Baidal, J.A., Locks, L.M., Cheng, E.R. et al. (2016). Risk factors for childhood obesity in the first 1,000 days: a systematic review. *Am. J. Prev. Med.* 50: 761–779.

60 Singhal, A. and Lucas, A. (2004). Early origins of cardiovascular disease: is there a unifying hypothesis? *Lancet* 363: 1642–1645.

61 Ong, K.K. and Loos, R.J. (2006). Rapid infancy weight gain and subsequent obesity: systematic reviews and hopeful suggestions. *Acta Paediatr.* 95: 904–908.

62 Singhal, A. (2016). The role of infant nutrition in the global epidemic of non-communicable disease. *Proc. Nutr. Soc.* 75: 162–168.

63 World Health Organization (2023). New WHO framework available for prevention and management of obesity. `https://www.who.int/news/item/17-05-2023-new-WHO-framework-available-for-prevention-and-management-of-obesity` (accessed 13 July 2023).

64 Brown, T., Moore, T.H., Hooper, L. et al. (2019). Interventions for preventing obesity in children. *Cochrane Database Syst. Rev.* 7: CD001871.

65 Lanigan, J., Collins, S., Birbara, T. et al. (2013). The TrimTots programme for prevention and treatment of obesity in preschool children: evidence from two randomised controlled trials. *Lancet* 382 (Suppl): 58.

10 Family Meal Times

Judith Cruikshank and Laura Stewart

'Getting to the heart of what is causing the eating habits'. [1]

Introduction

Family mealtimes are portrayed as the whole family sitting together around a dining table, where everyone is enjoying the same meal and participating in positive social interactions. This expectation of what a family mealtime should look like however is not the reality for a lot of families, and there can be a number of reasons as to why.

In today's world, family dynamics can be different to what they were in previous decades. In many of today's households one or both parents work, adding to time pressures at the end of the day to prepare family meals. A family home may not have the space for a large enough dining table for everyone to sit around at the same time, or indeed any table at all. This can result in individuals eating at different times or being spread out to eat in various parts of the home. Meals may be taken while watching television or using a computer or other electronic device. In families where there are younger children, they may eat earlier in the evening and adult(s) later after child's bedtime routine.

As well as some general logistical issues within homes, there can also be the issue of 'fussy eaters' resulting in different meals being prepared. Different meals being prepared can be stressful and often result in tension or arguments. The preparation of multiple meals can occur whether individuals ultimately eat altogether or separately.

A chapter on this subject is an important part of a textbook on the topic of childhood obesity. Parents will describe issues around meal and snack times, with the struggle to cope with family and individual behaviours

Child and Adolescent Obesity: A Practical Approach to Clinical Weight Management,
First Edition. Edited by Laura Stewart.
© 2024 John Wiley & Sons Ltd. Published 2024 by John Wiley & Sons Ltd.

around food at times feeling like an almost insurmountable problem. Many parents attending a childhood weight management clinic will describe their child as being a 'fussy eater'. Therefore, this chapter aims to outline how parent and child behaviour can be changed and strategies implemented to facilitate calm family mealtimes, alleviating stress and pressure, and ensuring the family mealtime environment is optimised.

Benefits of Family Mealtimes

Having a meal with someone can help nurture an individual's development and studies have shown that family mealtimes are linked to better nutrition and can be a predictor for success in life [2]. A review undertaken on the promotion of family meals found evidence suggesting '*regular family meals protect against unhealthy eating and obesity during childhood and adolescence*' [3]. Participating in mealtimes with at least one other person encourages behaviours such as communication and social skills. In fact, the behaviour of eating together can lead to social sustenance and these skills can then be transferred into a wider range of familiar environments (such as school canteens, cafes, and restaurants), and give individuals the confidence to enter unfamiliar environments which they have previously avoided.

Family mealtimes provide opportunities for children to build on their communication and social skills and can start from an early age when the parent(s) sit and chat while feeding, continuing to build on this as the child gets older and are eating independently. For example, sitting together having a family meal and recalling what has happened during their day at nursery, school, after school clubs etc. or discussing and planning weekend activities. It does not always have to be a formal family meal for social and communication skills to be learnt, it can also be while parent sits having a coffee as their child has a snack or meal.

Another benefit of family mealtimes is eating shared meals. It is more cost effective for the whole family to be eating the same meals. Shared meals eliminate the requirement to prepare different foods for one mealtime, but sometimes different foods are offered to avoid confrontation and potential refusal to eat. Preparing a shared meal takes less preparation time, is cost effective and can help promote family eating balanced meals. This is evidenced in the cross-sectional study by Ducrot et al. who showed that by planning ahead individuals had an increased food variety and better dietary quality [4].

Fussy Eating

Also referred to as picky or selective, fussy eating is an unwillingness to eat unfamiliar foods or to try new foods, as well as having strong food preferences often resulting in poor dietary variety from childhood [5].

Often beginning in early toddler years, and sometimes 'out the blue' children can develop fussy eating behaviours. Although some parents expect this and for their child to grow out of it, sometimes the fussy eating continues as the child gets older [6]. However, studies have shown that healthy eating in childhood can lead to a continuation of this behaviour into adulthood, helping individuals avoid health issues in later life [7]. Children can learn behaviour by observing and modelling others, so parental eating behaviour and their own food preferences can be influential and provide opportunities to model good eating habits [8].

Behaviour

What do we mean when we speak about behaviour? Often the first thought would be someone's negative or problematic actions that are causing disruption. However, from a behavioural perspective, human behaviour is made up of everything that a person does from what they say and what they do and depends on the environment in which it occurs [9]. Both social and physical settings within an environment are responsible for people's behaviour.

Figure 10.1 shows a simplified pathway of the ABC of contingency behaviour modification. The antecedent triggers a person to respond to their environment (behaviour) and as a result there is a subsequent change in the environment (consequence). This change may be immediate, or it may occur after a period of time.

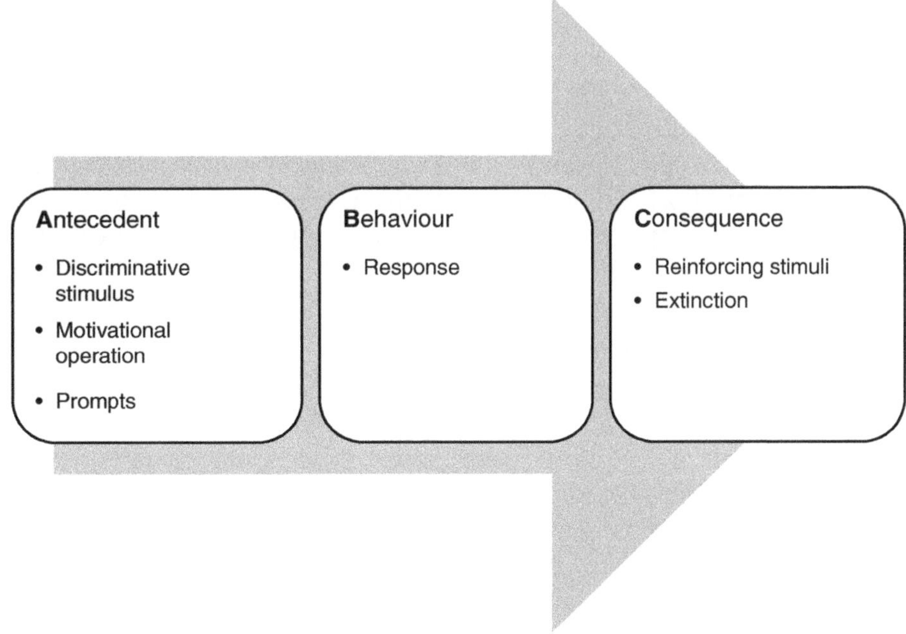

Figure 10.1 Three-term contingency of behaviour modification.

The Antecedent

An antecedent is a stimulus change that occurs within the environment immediately before the behaviour and can signal the availability of reinforcement. The discriminative stimuli (S^D) can be anything that an individual sees, hears, tastes, smells, or touches within their environment. For example, when you hear someone say 'time for lunch' you will do a set of behaviours you have previously undertaken prior to receiving lunch, for example washing your hands and then going and sitting down where lunch is usually provided.

Another antecedent to our behaviour is motivational operations (MOs) which are environmental conditions or events that temporarily increase or decrease the value (desire) of some stimulus as a consequence. The two common MOs are deprivation and satiation. Deprivation will increase the value of a reinforcer which has been unavailable for a specific period and evoke behaviour that has resulted in access to these items in the past. Satiation on the other hand has the opposite effect and will decrease the value of a reinforcer as it has been freely available [10].

When learning any new behaviour, assistance can be provided through the form of prompts. Prompting used as an antecedent can assist with the correct behaviour (response) being emitted and can take the form of for example hand-over-hand prompting, modelling, visual cues, and gesture prompts (glances or pointing).

Consequence

A consequence is a stimulus change that occurs after target behaviour and influences future behaviour. Two such consequences utilised within a behavioural approach are reinforcement and extinction. Reinforcement occurs after a response, and that response is then more likely or equally likely to occur again in the future under similar situations [11, 12], showing that the behaviour is either increased or maintained by reinforcement. Extinction also occurs as a consequence and therefore after a response and is used to decrease the frequency of a target behaviour [13]. Consequences that are combined with an antecedent condition will result in learning.

An everyday example of the three-term contingency (or what is sometimes referred to as the A-B-Cs of behaviour) would be where a child is hungry (MO/antecedent) and asks for a biscuit (behaviour) and is then given a biscuit (consequence). The way in which the child initially asked for the biscuit was reinforced (as the child was given a biscuit) and therefore the next time they are hungry and would like a biscuit they will undertake the same requesting behaviour that resulted in them getting the biscuit previously.

Manipulation of antecedents and consequences can alter behaviour and will be discussed later under Strategies section.

Parenting Styles

The process of raising a child is referred to as parenting and it comes with the responsibility of *'providing them with protection and care in order to ensure their healthy development into adulthood'* [14]. This includes the social, emotional, and physical support they require.

A ground-breaking study in the early 1970s by Diana Baumrind identified two dimensions of parents' behaviour which, when combined, revealed parenting styles. Baumrind originally combined the dimensions of responsiveness and structured expectations which created three main parenting styles: authoritarian, permissive and authoritative, with the latter being *'found to be the more ideal parenting style, leading to more positive cognitive, social, and emotional development in children and adolescents'*. [15]

Since the pioneering work of Baumrind, decades of research has taken place replicating the findings of this research and further developing our understanding of parental styles. There are now understood to be four main types of parenting styles: authoritarian, permissive, neglectful/uninvolved, and authoritative [16].

Authoritarian parenting style has characteristics of low responsiveness and high demandingness, often with one-way communication where the parent enforces strict rules that should be followed regardless of the child's feelings or objections – parents might say things such as 'because I said so'. In a study by Rhee, Lumeng, Appugliese et al. *'authoritarian parenting was associated with the highest risk of overweight among young children'* [17] and in the study conducted by Diabetes.co.uk it was found that children of authoritarian parenting were linked to higher weight gain [18].

The permissive parenting style has high responsiveness and low demandingness traits. Any rules set by parents are rarely enforced and little direction is given, allowing children to make their own decisions. With this style of parenting, the parent is more lenient and conflict is often avoided. Often grandparents use permissive parenting style where they provide little rules and see their role as having permission to spoil their grandchild [19].

The neglectful (or sometimes referred to as uninvolved) parenting style has low responsiveness and low demandingness. With this style parents do not spend time with their child so do not know where they are or what they are doing. There can be very little rules within the household and little guidance, attention and nurturing provided by the parent.

Authoritative parenting style has common traits of high responsiveness and high demandingness, parents spend time and effort creating and maintaining a positive relationship with their child, nurturing them, and taking into consideration their feelings and opinions. Rules are set with a degree of flexibility built in.

Studies by Zeltser and Liem et al., to name two, have shown that the authoritative parenting approach is the most effective in raising socially competent, self-reliant, and independent children within Western cultures [16, 20]. Authoritative parenting has also been shown to assist weight management. Children from parents adopting permissive and neglectful parenting style *'were twice as likely to be overweight, compared with children of authoritative mothers'* [17] and in a review undertaken by Sokol et al. it found authoritative parenting to be associated with lower risk of obesity and BMI gains [21].

Further supporting the authoritative parenting style is The Triple P – Positive Parenting Program – which is an evidence-based parenting programme implemented across the world. Developed by Professor Matt Sanders and colleagues at the University of Queensland in Australia, the programme provides parents with the tools to build a stronger family structure while addressing the emotional and behavioural problems faced by their children [22].

When asked which parental style to use, there is not one style that will fit all situations and it is about parents adopting the best style in certain family situations. For example, an authoritative parent may adopt permissive traits when their child is unwell (providing more sweets or fizzy juice than normal) and a permissive parent may enforce an authoritative trait of strict rules where safety becomes important.

Although an effective style of parenting within Europe and America, Febiyanti and Rachmawati found that authoritative parenting style may not be as effective in Asian countries and *'the meaning of the best parenting style tends to be influenced by the norms and values in the respective culture'* [23].

Strategies

In order to achieve the goal of establishing or increasing family mealtimes, there are a number of strategies that a professional working in weight management can consider. These all involve changing the existing behaviours around mealtimes of both the parent and the child. The information below is an outline of suggested strategies and should only be used as a guide.

Considerations Prior to Implementing a Strategy

Prior to implementing behaviour strategy, any potential health issues need to be ruled out first. This is very important, and any behavioural approach should only be implemented once there is certainty that medical issues are not playing a part in an individual's behaviour. Time also needs to be taken into consideration prior to implementing a strategy. This not only refers to the time to set things up but also the potential time it will take for any strategy to take effect on the target behaviour. Any targeted behaviour change may not have a 'quick fix'. Another key consideration prior to implementing any strategy is ensuring everyone who has contact with the child is on board with the strategy, for example immediate and extended family members, teachers etc. The lead parent does not want to spend time and effort implementing a strategy for someone in the child's kinship circle to then undo all their hard work. This can be particularly true of grandparents, who may treat children differently to parents and can be seen as disruptors to plans. A study by Eli et al. in 2016 found that some grandparents reported their role as '*holding certain "privileges" and having the right to "spoil" grandchildren with "treats" as part of grandparenting*' [24]. Grandparents' permissiveness may cause problems, so it is important to highlight this at an early planning stage and speak to them and explain the importance of following the strategy that is being put in place.

Antecedent-based Strategies

Antecedent strategies '*are put in place with the goal of preventing a behaviour from occurring in the first place*' [12] and a strategy often utilised by authoritative parents [25]. Example antecedent strategies are managing appetite, providing choices, and modelling.

Research has shown that children of permissive parents are more likely to develop health problems, such as obesity, as they struggle to promote exercise and limit unhealthy foods [25]. Snacking is the behaviour of consuming food in between meals; however, these 'snacks' are often nutrient-poor and energy-dense foods and evidence shows that children who frequently snack have poorer diet quality and consume more energy which can lead to excessive weight gain [26]. Being concerned about a child's fussy eating behaviour often leads to them being allowed to graze and snack throughout the day with parents feeling that 'something is better than nothing'. However, this snacking behaviour can make it difficult to manage a child's appetite and ultimately makes family mealtimes even more problematic. In order to manage the child's appetite, good practice would be to minimise unhealthy snacking during the day – perhaps a small healthy snack in the morning and/or the afternoon, thus increasing appetite for family mealtimes.

The physical and social environmental context of mealtimes can play a part in dietary behaviours, and meal planning and structure, such as eating as a family, can be effective strategies. A structure around mealtime, such as not eating in front of the television and eating an evening meal at a routine time, has been shown to assist children to eat a higher-quality diet, particularly by authoritative parents. In the same study lower mealtime structure was evident in authoritarian parenting style and resulted in children having a lower dietary quality [27]. A structure around mealtime can also assist with anxiety. If children know what to expect, then they can better understand what is expected of them [2].

Meal planning, the act of planning food and meals for the coming days, is regarded as good practice in terms of saving time and money. Buying only what is needed also results in less food wastage, ultimately helping the environment. An investigation into whether there is an association between diet quality and meal planning showed that *'individuals planning their meals were more likely to have a better dietary quality, including a higher adherence with nutritional guidelines as well as an increased food variety'* [4]

Providing choices as an antecedent strategy has been shown to decrease problem behaviours at mealtimes and increase the amount of healthy food eaten by individuals. Increasing the choice on offer has the effect of increasing the likelihood that the individual will like at least one of the choices presented [28]. Earlier in the chapter, the term 'satiation' was mentioned in relation to the effect it has on motivation. When referring to food, satiation can have the effect of reducing the desire to eat some or all of a preferred item. For example, if you have the same item of food for breakfast (e.g., toast) for a long period you will get tired of eating this food. Providing choices, such as toast, cereals, and fruit, allows for an individual to eat more of the choices presented and will move to eating the new items when had enough of the toast.

Previously, Figure 10.1 showed that prompting appeared under the antecedent heading. Modelling is a form of prompting and is a useful antecedent strategy that involves observing another person. Decades of research has been undertaken looking at the effects of modelling on diet. Authoritative parenting style predicts greater use of parent modelling of healthy eating, which is the opposite of permissive and authoritarian parenting which uses less modelling of healthy eating [27]. The availability of healthy food within the household and modelling the eating of these foods are both predictors of healthier diets in children over time [29]. An important social factor is parental role modelling of healthy eating behaviours and correlates with children's preferences and intake of vegetables and fruits. Research has shown that children learn through observing the behaviours of others, including their peers and parents. Therefore, it is important to ensure that parental role modelling is an active and continual process at both mealtimes and snacks. This will encourage greater consumption of fruits, vegetables, and lower energy snacks [30].

Consequence-based Strategies

This type of strategy is key to overall behaviour change as it has the effect of strengthening and maintaining a behaviour (reinforcement) or decreasing the frequency of a behaviour (extinction). Positive reinforcement, planned ignoring, and token economies are examples of consequence-based strategies.

As mentioned earlier under the section on 'Behaviour', reinforcement occurs after a response (behaviour) and that behaviour is then more likely or equally likely to occur in the future under similar situations. Reinforcement can be positive or negative. Positive reinforcement is *'anything that is <u>added</u> to the environment after a behaviour that <u>increases</u> the likelihood of that behaviour recurring under similar circumstances'* and conversely negative reinforcement is *'anything <u>removed</u> from the environment after a behaviour that <u>increases</u> the likelihood of that behaviour recurring under similar circumstances'* [11].

A reinforcer, sometimes also referred to as an incentive or reward, is anything that acts as reinforcement for an individual. What is reinforcing for one individual may not be reinforcing for another. Examples of natural unconditioned reinforcers are water and food (thirst and hunger) which everyone needs in order to survive. Secondary or conditioned reinforcers are things such as verbal praise or compliments, books, toys, money, favourite foods etc. These items become reinforcing through exposure and contact/interaction with them. Using reinforcers is a powerful means of achieving behaviour change but only if used correctly. It must ensure that what is reinforcing for the individual has been accurately assessed, and this can be achieved by observing what they do and what they interact with. Reinforcers must only be provided when the target behaviour is happening (i.e., the reinforcer is contingent on target behaviour being observed) and the correct amount made available in order to motivate the individual to undertake the desired target behaviour. Varying the amount of reinforcement is called differential reinforcement and is used to ensure that greater reinforcement is provided to the individual for appropriate target behaviour than when they display the problem behaviour [12].

The use of positive reinforcement is the most common element of any intervention used to address healthy eating habits, where an individual will be given access to a reinforcer for engaging in a specific behaviour (i.e., trying a new food). One example of this is the 'Kids Choice' lunch programme that was implemented to encourage children in an elementary school to accept fruits and vegetables. By providing tokens as a form of positive reinforcement, the study showed that this had a positive impact on increasing not only fruit and vegetable intake but also the children's enjoyment of these items compared to individuals who did not take part in the intervention [31].

Token economy systems are a useful reinforcement strategy, but rather than providing immediate reinforcement there is a time delay in the individual gaining access to their reward (reinforcement). There are three components to a token economy, the tokens (which can take the form of objects such as stickers, stamps etc.), the reinforcer (which is the object or activity that the individual values) and the exchange (which occurs when the earned tokens are exchanged for access to the desired reinforcer).

Extinction is used to decrease the frequency of negative behaviours, and the active process of planned ignoring is one way of achieving this. During mealtimes if reinforcement in any form (e.g., attention) has previously been given for negative behaviour (such as spitting food out or refusing to eat), this attention needs to stop so the spitting out food and refusal to eat would be ignored. On some occasions the negative behaviour may actually increase prior to reducing which is referred to as the extinction burst. Using positive reinforcement during mealtimes requires not only ignoring the negative behaviours but also paying attention to the appropriate behaviours (e.g., using utensils, eating food you have offered) [32]. Extinction does not always provide a 'quick fix', so it is important that everyone adheres to the plan of implementing planned ignoring – everyone ignores any inappropriate behaviour, for example whining at mealtime to gain access to a sugary drink and ensuring they provide praise for the target behaviour such as eating a new food. This takes practice and patience but will result in positive behaviour from the individual.

It is important to highlight here that bribery is not the same as positive reinforcement. Bribery is defined in dictionaries as persuading another to act improperly which is not what reinforcement is setting out to do – it has the effect of making a positive change to individuals healthy eating habits.

Further detailed information on strategies to use with fussy eaters can be found in the useful book called *Broccoli Boot Camp* by Drs Williams and Seiverling [28].

Further Considerations

Increasing Foods: Diet Variety

Regular meals which assist in the regulation of sugar and eating a varied diet which provides necessary nutrients to support the brain are both required by children in order to facilitate good mood, behaviour, and learning [33]. As human beings, we are not born knowing what foods we like and dislike, these are learned through exposure to foods (conditioned reinforcer) and tasting from early childhood. Smith and colleagues found a link between food fussiness (being selective about food choices due to attributes such as texture) and food neophobia which refers to the refusal to try unfamiliar foods. They suggest that familial and home environments play a more important role in shaping food fussiness than food neophobia in early years [34]. A number of other studies have shown that repeated taste exposure and taste-based conditioning strategies assist in increasing vegetable consumption [35, 36] and diet variety. Many parents give up after the child has had only one or two exposures to a new food and do not persist enough with taste exposure to make a difference to new food preferences. A review by Nekitsing and colleagues found that a minimum of 8–10 repeated taste exposures are required before a new taste preference may be developed [37].

Likes versus Dislikes

It is not uncommon to hear phrases such as 'yuck' when children are presented with a new food, with them making a judgement (often on how it looks) before tasting has even taken place. Only through taste exposure can a decision be made as to whether they truly 'like' or 'dislike' specific items of food. If the individual is older a list of those foods they like and those they do not like can be produced, after taste exposure has taken place.

Some good practice to adopt would be to show children where food comes from and also participate in food preparation. Going shopping together and exposing them to various foods and allowing them to participate in the preparation of the meals can all assist in reducing the resistance to trying new foods. Children who are too young to help with preparation could be sitting in the same room to observe the food preparation and allow parents to talk to them and provide social interaction during the process. Another good practice would be to play board games that involve food and also play with pretend food items to get them used to handling different foods.

Portion Sizes

Many parents are concerned about making sure their child eats enough, but good practice would be to concentrate on quality of diet rather than quantity of food intake. In order to provide a balanced diet, meals should be made up of items from all food groups, which the Eatwell Guide outlines as five portions of fruits and vegetables, carbohydrates (e.g. potatoes, bread, rice, pasta), dairy and calcium, proteins (e.g. beans, pulses, fish, eggs, meat), and six to eight cups of water per day. This guide is aimed at individuals from the age of 2 years and older [33].

Measuring Progress

A behavioural approach uses data to assess behaviour change and make a decision as to whether strategies that are currently in place are effective or not in reaching the target behaviour. Data can also be used to make decisions such as how and when to make alterations to existing strategy and whether or not to move to a different intervention. Prior to implementing a new strategy, it is recommended that all current conditions such as existing foods individual will eat and any types of negative behaviour they currently display when offered new foods are recorded. This information is referred to as the baseline. The baseline is then assessed against future data once strategies are implemented to evaluate any changes that have occurred in the individual's behaviour (e.g., has intake of new foods occurred). Information can be recorded in items such as diaries, and against meal plans.

Autism Spectrum Disorder and Other Developmental Disorders

Parents of children with a diagnosis of autism and other developmental disorders often raise the question about how to improve their child's diet. Many children with a diagnosis such as autism spectrum disorder (ASD), attention-deficit/hyperactive disorder (ADHD), anxiety and depression are fussy eaters and have a limited nutritional diet with the main food intake for individuals with ASD appearing to focus on, for example, crunchy foods, white foods and carbohydrates. Fussy eating in individuals with obesity and a disorder including ADHD, ASD, anxiety or depression was the focus of a study by Thornsteinsdottir and colleagues who found that fussy eating was greater among children with anxiety and obesity [38].

The A-B-Cs of behaviour and strategies outlined earlier in the chapter can be applied to individuals with ASD and other developmental disorders. Consideration should also be given to sensory issues, so additional preparation may require to be undertaken prior to implementation of a strategy. Sensory processing and behaviour issues around mealtimes was the focus of a recent synthesis of studies which found support for a significant relationship between a broad range of eating behaviours and sensory processing in autism [39]. Considering sensory input, good practice would be to look at ensuring no identifying marks on bowls, cups etc. so that individuals do not become dependent on them and therefore only being able to eat or drink from these specific items. Keeping items neutral will also assist individuals in transitioning to eating in restaurants, school canteens, cafes etc.

Conclusions

Through the use of antecedent and consequence-based strategies, parent and child behaviour can be changed in order to facilitate family mealtimes, alleviating any stress and pressure and ensuring the family mealtime environment is optimised.

WHAT DOES THIS MEAN IN PRACTICE?

- Consider the existing patenting style and culture within the family home.
- Undertake an assessment of existing family mealtime issue.
- Identified target behaviours to be addressed.
- Implement the agreed strategy in small achievable steps, ensuring all involved are signed up to it.
- Assess existing strategy to measure its effectiveness, making any necessary changes.

References

1 Stewart, L. (2022). Personal communication:practitioner.
2 Rowell, K. and McGlothlin, J. (2015). *Helping Your Child with Extreme Picky Eating: A Step-by Step Guide for Overcoming Selective Eating, Food Aversion, and Feeding Disorders*. New Harbinger Publications, Inc.
3 Hennessy, E., Dwyer, L., Oh, A. et al. (2015). Promoting family meals: a review of existing interventions and opportunities for future research. *Adolesc. Health Med. Ther.* 115: https://doi.org/10.2147/ahmt.s37316.
4 Ducrot, P., Méjean, C., Aroumougame, V. et al. (2017). Meal planning is associated with food variety, diet quality and body weight status in a large sample of French adults. *Int. J. Behav. Nutr. Phys. Act.* 14: https://doi.org/10.1186/s12966-017-0461-7.
5 Taylor, C.M., Wernimont, S.M., Northstone, K. et al. (2015). Picky/fussy eating in children: review of definitions, assessment, prevalence and dietary intakes. *Appetite* 95: 349–359. https://doi.org/10.1016/j.appet.2015.07.026.
6 Wolstenholme, H., Kelly, C., Hennessy, M. et al. (2020). Childhood fussy/picky eating behaviours: a systematic review and synthesis of qualitative studies. *Int. J. Behav. Nutr. Phys. Act.* 17: https://doi.org/10.1186/s12966-019-0899-x.
7 Lim, G.W. and Shin, K.M. (2022). The influence of parental eating behaviors, child-feeding practices, and infants' temperaments upon infants' eating behaviors. *Clin. Exp. Pediatr.* 65: 466–468. https://doi.org/10.3345/cep.2021.01865.

8   Scaglioni, S., Salvioni, M., and Galimberti, C. (2008). Influence of parental attitudes in the development of children eating behaviour. *Br. J. Nutr.* 29: https://doi.org/10.1017/S0007114508892471.

9   Saarloos, D., Kim, J.-E., and Timmermans, H. (2009). The built environment and health: introducing individual space-time behavior. *Int. J. Environ. Res. Public Health* 6: 1724–1743. https://doi.org/10.3390/ijerph6061724.

10 Barbera, M.L. (2007). *The Verbal Behavior Approach: How to Teach Children with Autism and Related Disorders*. Jessica Kingsley Publishers.

11 Schramm, R. (2006). *Educate Towards Recovery: Turning the Tables on Autism – a Teaching Manual for the Verbal Behavior Approach to ABA*. Lulu.

12 Glasberg, B.A. (2008). *STOP that Seemingly Senseless Behavior! FBA-based Interventions for People with Autism*, 1e. Woodbine House, Inc.

13 Kearney, A.J. (2008). *Understanding Applied Behavior Analysis: An Introduction to ABA for Parents, Teachers, and other Professionals*. Jessica Kingsley Publishers.

14 Kretchmar-Hendricks, M. (2023). Parenting. https://www.britannica.com/topic/parenting (accessed 12 February 2023).

15 Cowan, P.A. (2020). In memoriam Diana B Baumrind. https://senate.universityofcalifornia.edu/in-memoriam/files/diana-baumrind.html (accessed 31 January 2023).

16 Zeltser F. (2021). A psychologist shares the 4 styles of parenting – and the type that researchers say is the most successful. https://www.cnbc.com/2021/06/29/child-psychologist-explains-4-types-of-parenting-and-how-to-tell-which-is-right-for-you.html (accessed 31 January 2023).

17 Rhee, K.E., Lumeng, J.C., Appugliese, D.P. et al. (2006). Parenting styles and overweight status in first grade. *Pediatrics* 117: 2047–2054. https://doi.org/10.1542/peds.2005-2259.

18 Diabetes.co.uk (2022). Children with stricter parents are more likely to grow up obese. https://www.diabetes.co.uk/news/2022/oct/children-with-stricter-parents-are-more-likely-to-grow-up-obese-study-finds.html (accessed 31 January 2023).

19 Team Beenke (2023). Dealing with permissive grandparents. https://beenke.com/health-relationship/dealing-permissive-grandparents/ (accessed 1 February 2023).

20 Liem, J.H., Cavell, E.C., and Lustig, K. (2010). The influence of authoritative parenting during adolescence on depressive symptoms in young adulthood: examining the mediating roles of self-development and peer support. *J. Genet. Psychol.* 171: 73–92. https://doi.org/10.1080/00221320903300379.

21 Sokol, R.L., Qin, B., and Poti, J.M. (2017). Parenting styles and body mass index: a systematic review of prospective studies among children. *Obes. Rev.* 18: 281–292. https://doi.org/10.1111/obr.12497.

22 Professor Sanders, M. (2023). Triple P. https://www.triplep.net/glo-en/home/ (accessed 14 February 2023).

23 Febiyanti, A. and Rachmawati, Y. (2021. http://doi.org/10.2991/assehr.k.210322.021). *Is Authoritative Parenting the Best Parenting Style?* Atlantis Press.

24 Eli, K., Howell, K., Fisher, P.A. et al. (2016). A question of balance: explaining differences between parental and grandparental perspectives on preschoolers' feeding and physical activity. *Soc. Sci. Med.* 154: 28–35. https://doi.org/10.1016/j.socscimed.

25 Morin, A. (2022). The 4 types of parenting styles and how kids are affected. Very well family. https://www.verywellfamily.com/types-of-parenting-styles-1095045 (accessed 23 February 2023).

26 Blaine, R.E., Kachurak, A., Davison, K.K. et al. (2017). Food parenting and child snacking: a systematic review. *Int. J. Behav. Nutr. Phys. Act.* 14: https://doi.org/10.1186/s12966-017-0593-9.

27 Lopez, N.V., Schembre, S., Belcher, B.R. et al. (2018). Parenting styles, food-related parenting practices, and children's healthy eating: a meditation analysis to examine relationships between parenting and child diet. *Appetite* 128: 205–213. https://doi.org/10.1016/j.appet.2018.06.021.

28 Williams, K.E. and Seiverling, L.J. (2022). *Broccoli Boot Camp Basic Training for Parents of Selective Eaters*. AAPC Publishing.

29 Ventura, A.K. and Birch, L.L. (2008). Does parenting affect children's eating and weight status? *Int. J. Behav. Nutr. Phys. Act.* 5: 15. https://doi.org/10.1186/1479-5868-5-15.

30 Draxten, M., Fulkerson, J.A., Friend, S. et al. (2014). Parental role modeling of fruits and vegetables at meals and snacks is associated with children's adequate consumption. *Appetite* 78: 1–7. https://doi.org/10.1016/j.appet.2014.02.017.

31 Hendy, H.M., Williams, K.E., and Camise, T.S. (2005). Kids Choice' School lunch program increases children's fruit and vegetable acceptance. *Appetite* 45: 250–263. https://doi.org/10.1016/j.appet.2005.07.006.

32 Fraker, C., Fishbein, M., Cox, S. et al. (2007). *Food Chaining: The Proven 6-step Plan to Stop Picky Eating, Solve Feeding Problems, and Expand your Child's Diet*. Marlowe & Company.

33 BDA The Association of UK Dieticians (2023). Food fact sheet: diet, behaviour and learning in children. https://www.bda.uk.com/resource/diet-behaviour-and-learning-children.html (accessed 31 January 2023).

34 Smith, A.D., Herle, M., Fildes, A. et al. (2017). Food fussiness and food neophobia share a common etiology in early childhood. *J. Child Psychol. Psychiatry* 58: 189–196. https://doi.org/10.1111/jcpp.12647.

35 Appleton, K.M., Hemingway, A., Rajska, J. et al. (2018). Repeated exposure and conditioning strategies for increasing vegetable liking and intake: systematic review and meta-analyses of the published literature. *Am. J. Clin. Nutr.* 108: 842–856. https://doi.org/10.1093/ajcn/nqy143.

36 Karagiannaki, K., Ritz, C., Jensen, L.G.H. et al. (2021). Optimising repeated exposure: determining optimal exposure frequency for introducing a novel vegetable among children. *Foods* 10: 913. https://doi.org/10.3390/foods10050913.

37 Nekitsing, C., Blundell-Birtill, P., Cockroft, J.E. et al. (2018). Systematic review and meta-analysis of strategies to increase vegetable consumption in preschool children aged 2–5 years. *Appetite* 127: 138–154. https://doi.org/10.1016/j.appet.2018.04.019.

38 Thorsteinsdottir, S., Olafsdottir, A.S., Brynjolfsdottir, B. et al. (2022). Odds of fussy eating are greater among children with obesity and anxiety. *Obes. Sci. Pract.* 8: 91–100. https://doi.org/10.1002/osp4.548.

39 Nimbley, E., Golds, L., Sharpe, H. et al. (2022). Sensory processing and eating behaviours in autism: a systematic review. *Eur. Eat. Disord. Rev.* 30: 538–559. https://doi.org/10.1002/erv.2920.

11 Childhood Weight Management in Practice

Laura Stewart

'What you have done is give me back my happy smiley girl' [1]

Introduction

Throughout this book aspects of childhood obesity and its management have been explored. The aim of this chapter is to bring together components of previous discussions to give a practical overview on the delivery of weight management programmes. While many, if not all, of the aspects discussed will be relevant to any age group, in the first part of this chapter particular reference will be made to using programmes and programme components in the primary years age group (circa five to eleven years old). This part is rounded off with a case study of 10-year-old Daisy.

The chapter then moves on to consider treatment options to supplement lifestyle management, which are typically offered to young people 12 years and older. First, briefly looking at bariatric surgery and its place in any pathway of care for CYP, particularly adolescents living in the severe obesity range. Finally, the chapter concludes by considering the emerging role of next-generation pharmacology in the management of childhood obesity. This is still early days and will certainly be an area of much discussion over the coming years.

Service Structure

Previous chapters have considered essential aspects of a childhood weight management programme and the recommendations of evidenced-based guidelines [2, 3]. These have included:

- the appropriate use of language
- a non-stigmatising person-centred approach

Child and Adolescent Obesity: A Practical Approach to Clinical Weight Management,
First Edition. Edited by Laura Stewart.
© 2024 John Wiley & Sons Ltd. Published 2024 by John Wiley & Sons Ltd.

- the use of behavioural change tools
- lifestyle changes to dietary intake, physical activity and sedentary levels.

However, the guidelines do not describe the practical manner in which the components come together and fit into an overall comprehensive, family orientated, weight management programme. All these facets are brought together through this chapter in describing approaches to deliver childhood weight management programmes.

How a programme will be developed and delivered will be hugely dependant on the healthcare system in which it sits, the professionals delivering, the age of the CYP as well as the values and beliefs of the population in which it is being delivered. As an example of points to consider in a service development, Public Health Scotland (PHS) in 2019 published standards for the delivery of weight management service for CYP, these include:

- each area/region should have an explicit weight management pathway for CYP living with obesity
- on receiving a referral, a service should have a defined triage process which is taken on by an appropriately trained member of the team
- concerns regarding well-being and risk of harm are escalated appropriately (see Chapter 14)
- the mental well-being of the CYP should always be a consideration
- supported physical activity sessions should be a core component of the weight management programme
- weight management programmes should have a minimum of eight sessions – whether individual or group
- sessions should ideally be weekly or fortnightly
- post completion of the core programme on-going support should be offered [4].

Delivery Team

The 'gold standard' for programme delivery is by a specialist multidisciplinary childhood weight management team [2]. NHS England defines a multidisciplinary team (MDT) as:

> 'A multidisciplinary team (MDT) is a group of health and care staff who are members of different organisations and professions (e.g. GPs, social workers, nurses), that work together to make decisions regarding the treatment of individual patients and service users. MDTs are used in both health and care settings'.
> (Information sharing in Multidisciplinary Teams (MDTs) –
> NHS Transformation Directorate (england.nhs.uk) 2023).

A childhood weight management MDT could be composed in a variety of ways. It might include, but is not limited to, a combination of the following professionals:

- Dietitian (in some countries this may be a nutritionist)
- Psychologist
- Paediatrician – a general paediatrician or one specialising in diabetes or endocrinology
- Physiotherapist
- Nurse
- Social worker
- Family support worker
- Support worker
- Physical activity specialist
- Occupational therapist
- Youth worker

Regardless of the composition of the MDT, it should come together to regularly discuss the service development and day-to-day running of the programme. The team may meet and work with families together or in a number of profession combinations, i.e. the CYP and their parents may sit in a room with one member or multiply members of the MDT.

The MDT brings the sum of their clinical expertise and reasoning to working with the CYP and their families as well as to team discussions and debriefs. It is also an excellent opportunity to upskill all the professionals in the team, through in-action learning and intra MDT education lessons.

For the CYP and families, it provides them with a 'one stop shop' to have the input from a number of professionals. They have the opportunity to see the relevant professional without the need for onward referral and waiting times. A practical point would be to ensure that the CYP and parents are not overwhelmed or intimidated by a room full of professionals, making the appointment sessions too long or being continuingly asked the same questions by different members of the team. Therefore, there is a need for a well thought out patient journey through each clinical session and the overall programme.

Uni-profession Delivery

While delivery by an MDT is considered the 'gold standard', this will not always possible due to a number of reasons such as the historical delivery of healthcare in each country or region, budgets or the available of a range of professionals to take part. Therefore, it is not unusual for a service to be delivered or led by a uni-profession, i.e. one profession such as dietetics or medical physicians. When this does occur, what is important is that there are the resources available for discussion and onward referral to other teams and services, such as:

- Psychology and local child and adolescent mental health services (known in the UK as CAMHs)
- Paediatric endocrinologist or a consultant paediatrician with an interest in endocrinology
- Social worker
- Physical activity/leisure specialists

Programme Structure

Programmes tend to be delivered either as groups or as 1:1 sessions. There is a preference for 1:1 sessions for CYP when there are more complex medical and social requirements as well as for CYP with additional support needs. In the UK, community group childhood weight management is typically used for those CYP with lower BMIs, sometimes referred to as tier 2 services. While the 1:1 programmes are used for the CYP with higher BMIs, typically with a BMI $\geq$99.6th centile and particularly with complications of living with obesity. The better approach might be to have a mixture of both these within the same programme. Comparing group programmes with and without individual sessions, a review found there to be a better outcomes in BMI SD changes in the programmes with both group and individual sessions [5].

Without a doubt, a family approach is exceedingly important in supporting CYP weight management [6]. However, there are a number of programmes that take the approach of working solely and directly with the parents. The concept of targeting parents as the agents or mediators of change in childhood weight management was suggested by Golan in 2006 [7]. It is worth noting that a Cochrane (2015) review found that parent-only programmes had similar effects to parent and child programmes [8]. In practice, many programmes have parent-only aspects such as 1:1 programmes which include a number of parent-only sessions [9] and group programmes that have time with the parents and children together and then split into a parent-only group while typically the CYP have a physical activity session [10].

There are reports that programmes with more frequent contacts are more effective [11]. Public Health Scotland (PHS) have stated as essential in their standards of CYP weight management care that sessions should be delivered weekly or fortnightly and as essential that all interventions, groups or 1:1 have a minimum of eight sessions [4]. Indeed, a 2012 review by Ho et al. reported that better weight and BMI SD outcomes were seen when a programme was six months or longer [12].

Family Base Programme

All guidelines tell us that a programme should be family based. This makes perfect sense when considering the role adults play in modelling behaviour and how CYP imitate the behaviour of the adults around them. Behaviour change models such as the previously mentioned social cognitive theory (see Chapter 5) espouses an important tenet that the 'new' behaviour needs to be modelled to help the change take place. These points underpin why it is so important that any childhood weight management programme is designed and delivered in such a manner to include the parents and siblings. This should also include any significant adults in the kinship grouping who may take an active regular role in the family childcare arrangements such as grandparents. A situation to be avoided is, for example, one when a CYP has exchanged their after school snack from crisps to fruit while the rest of the family continue eating crisps prior to the evening meal. Therefore, throughout the process of the programme, it is imperative to emphasise the whole-family approach to behaviour change. This could include inviting the whole family to sessions as well as setting family-based lifestyle change goals.

There is evidence to suggest that family structures and dynamics can influence behaviour changes, either positively or negatively. One example of this is working with CYP who live in a blended family structure, i.e. the birth mother and father are not living together plus the possibility of a stepmother/father present with their own children. One of the birth parents may, for example, only see the CYP at alternative weeks or weekends. It is important to include all of the extended blended family. In reality, differing goals for lifestyle changes may need to be made for when staying with one or other of the parents due to differences in the values and commitment of the parents.

Assessment

An initial assessment session is the opportunity to start gathering and imparting information, this needs to be a two-way process. It is the point for starting to build rapport with the CYP and their parents [13]. This development of rapport and the two-way information sharing will continue as a process throughout the programme.

An initial parent-only session can be an exceedingly helpful way to allow the parents to express their concerns, opinions and thoughts about their child and their child's weight in a safe environment. When practiced as part of a routine programme structure, this initial parent-only session can be very informative.

A good assessment process will explore the holistic overview of the CYP's health and psycho-social well-being and family support structure [14, 15]. Clinical information and facts such as weight and BMI, weight history patterns, and previous attempts at weight control, comorbidities and any weight-related symptoms should be noted [16] along with:

- *'CYP's understanding of obesity*
- *Parents' understanding of obesity*
- *Potential barriers to change*
- *Current lifestyle: dietary intake, physical activity levels and time spent in sedentary behaviours*
- *Support networks, including extended family, school and friends*
- *Reward systems/strategies used to reinforce new behaviours'* [16].

Daisy – A Case Study

Programme Background

In the following case study, the BDA's Model and Process for Nutrition and Dietetic Practice (2016) is used as a template for recording the stages of the programme delivery and the clinical intervention's outcomes [17]. Figure 11.1 gives an outline of the stages of the BDA's Model and Process.

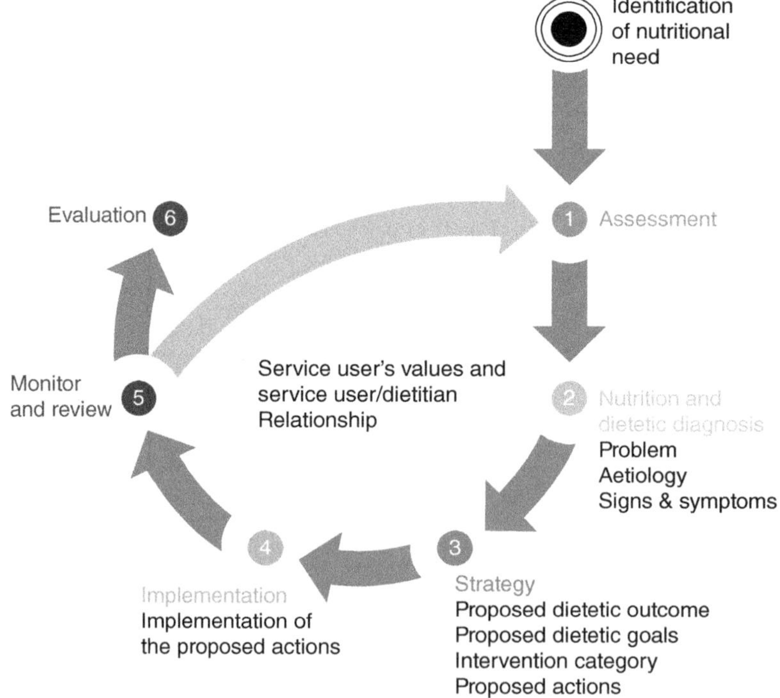

Figure 11.1 BDA model and process outline.

Source: Reproduced with permission from the British Dietetic Association (Oct 2023).

The programme used in the case study is the SCOTT programme based on a 1:1 intervention [9]. This was delivered by a dietetic-led childhood weight management team which included a dedicated clinical psychologist embedded in the team, as well as dietetic assistants specialising in family support and a team administrative assistant. The service had a formally agreed pathway and relationship with a paediatric consultant with an interest in endocrinology.

A service level agreement (SLA) was in place between the NHS weight management service and the local leisure company to deliver individual and support group physical activity sessions. This included six weekly bespoke 1:1 activity sessions for an hour with the CYP and their parents. These sessions were held locally and encouraged a range of family activities such as badminton, short tennis and swing ball. After the six individual family sessions, the family were then invited to group sessions for families to help encourage ongoing activities. A free family leisure pass for 12 months was given to families once they completed the six 1:1 activity sessions. This physical activity part of the programme was free to the families, being funded from the NHS's budget.

The programme was delivered as:

- **Session 1** – parent-only and lasting for up to one hour.
- **Session 2** – two weeks later with parents and Daisy for up to one hour.
- **Sessions 3 – 8** every 2 weeks for up to 30 minutes for Daisy and her parents. Siblings and other significant adults, for example grandparents, were also invited. Session 5 was set as parent only.
- **Sessions 9–10** every 4 weeks for up to 30 minutes.
- **Post programme**, a three-monthly review was offered as a session up to 30 minutes.

Identification of Nutritional Need

Daisy was 9 years and 10 months old when she was referred to the local NHS paediatric weight management team by her family GP.

Triage – The first stage of the service's triage and referral acceptance procedure was for the referral to be discussed and triaged by the whole team at the weekly team meeting and triage session. The team noted that Daisy's parents had attended the GP as they were concerned about her shortness of breath when running around. The GP had carried out a full examination and found no underlying cause for this shortness of breath. Daisy's parents said they were aware that she appeared to be larger than the other children in her Primary class. The GP asked if they wished to be referred to the service and they had agreed. Daisy's parents also said that she was shy and had few friends in or out of school.

A weight and height measurement was included in the referral. This was calculated to a BMI, which sat above the 99.6[th] BMI centile on the WHO/UK 1990 female BMI charts. Daisy was accepted as a referral onto the next stage of the service's triaging process.

Daisy's mother was then spoken to over the phone by an allocated member of the team. She indicated that both mum and dad were concerned about Daisy's recent and continuing weight gain. Although they mentioned being worried about her long-term health, their main concern was around her exceedingly small social group and her interactions with her peer group at school. Information detailing the outline of the programme involved was at that point posted out to the parents with an initial parent-only appointment time.

The time from the team receiving the referral to the date of the first session was 10 weeks.

Assessment

Anthropometry – Weight = 50 kg; Height = 1.30 m; At age 10 years the BMI = 29.6 sitting greater than the >99.6[th] centile, plotted on the WHO/UK 1990 female BMI charts. Waist:height ratio – 68/130 = 0.52, indicating increased health risks.

Biochemistry – None taken, as a dietetic-led service it was not usual practice to review biochemistry in childhood weight management unless there was an indication of underlying medical cause such as short stature or indication of a co-morbidity, for example if symptoms of type 2 diabetes were present.

Clinical – Clinical obesity due to BMI being above the 99.6[th] centile. No other medical history to note from the GP's letter or from a discussion with her parents.

Dietary – From a typical day dietary recall given by Daisy and supported by her parents she appeared to eat well-balanced meals. On discussion, these appeared to include excessively large portion sizes for age and her intake included multiple snacks between meals.

Environment – From a family social point of view, Daisy lived at home with her mother, father and younger brother. She was in her last year of primary school. She appeared to have little social contact with school peers either during school hours or outside of school. She did not attend any school or external clubs. Neither social work nor Children and Adolescent Mental Health team (CAMHs) were involved.

A SHANARRI assessment (see Chapter 14 for further details) indicated that she had:

- A supportive family
- Low self-esteem and confidence

- Excessive screen time
- Very low activity levels
- Making changes might be difficult for Daisy as her parents felt she might not be able to take responsibility to make changes outside the home.
- She had few friends and was being bullied at school due to her weight.

Focus – *Daisy* and her parents had attended the GP surgery due to mum's concerns that she had been getting progressively more overweight in the proceeding 2 years, including having put on 4 kg in the last month. Both parents were concerned about her weight gain but did not feel she had a particular 'unhealthy' dietary intake. She appeared at assessment stage to be sedentary, spending a lot of her day on screen time.

When explored over the first two sessions, motivation to change was recorded as:

Daisy – 8/10
Mother – 8/10

Discussions on *'what would be the good things about getting your weight under control'* elicited a list of:

- Will not be called names at school
- Will be able to run faster at PE
- Will make herself feel able to take part in school activities
- Will be able to get fashionable clothes

While exploring what she felt might be difficult about make changes (her barriers to change). Daisy and her parents gave a list of the following:

- Might feel hungry between meals
- Will be tired from any exercise
- Will miss watching favourite TV programme
- Will miss playing games on computer

Nutrition and Dietetic Diagnosis

Problem – childhood obesity.
Aetiology – sedentary lifestyle, excessive hunger with snacking on sweets.
Signs and symptoms – BMI above 99.6[th] centile, waist:height ratio 0.52, bullying.

Strategy

Daisy and her family were invited onto the SCOTT 1:1 family weight management programme. This included setting SMART lifestyle behaviour changes and reviewing these at subsequent sessions. The dietetic target was for Daisy to remain the same weight and, as a result of her increasing height, for this to show as a decrease in her BMI.

After the exploration of the family's motivation to change, they were given a lifestyle diary and asked to record Daisy's intake of food and drink, level of physical activity and screen time for the next two weeks until the following session.

Daisy and her family also agreed for a referral into the dedicated family physical activity programme delivered by the local leisure group for those in the childhood weight management service.

Implementation

Goal setting was introduced at Daisy's second session, which was actually the third appointment within the programme. Daisy and her parents' problem solved, agreed and set the following two goals:

- At least 20 minutes of activity three times per week
- Crisps after at evening meal no more than four times in a week

Monitor and Review

After attending 10 sessions over 6 months, Daisy had:

- Decreased her portion sizes at meal times by routinely using a smaller plate
- Stopped having crisps as snacks after school and only had fruits after coming home from school and after her evening meal
- Increase her physical activity to 30–60 minutes 5 days each week, she now attended the school hockey and football clubs
- Only had puddings at home on a Sunday
- Reduced her screen time to four to five hours six days per week

During the sessions, it was identified by the parents and the dietitian that the parents would benefit from some more information regarding reading food labels and on expanding their cooking skills. Mum subsequently went on a 1:1 supermarket session with the team's dietetic support worker and had three sessions with a local charity delivering family cooking skills.

Family changes included:

- Cooking smaller amounts of food to help with decreasing portion sizes
- Planning the weekly shopping list to help reduce the number of snacks in the house and to purchase more fruit and vegetables
- The whole family stopped eating crisps after the evening meal and instead had fruit
- As a family, they went swimming once a week and continued to attend the family-based group activities.

Weight $= 50.5\,$kg; Height $= 1.325$. At age 10 years and 6 months, the BMI $= 28.8$, sitting greater than the 99.6[th] centile, plotted on the WHO/UK 1990 female BMI charts. Waist:height ratio $- 68/1325 = 0.51$, increased health risks indicated.

Evaluation

Daisy and her family continued to attend the three-monthly follow-up sessions. At one year from initial referral, Daisy and her parents reported that she was actively involved in after-school clubs and regularly had sleep-overs with her friends. The family still went swimming together once a week and also continued to attend the family group activity sessions run by the leisure company. Her screen time was still lower than when she had started the programme as were her portion sizes and number of daily snacks.

Daisy's anthropometric measurements were:

Weight $= 50.5$ Height $= 1.36$. At age 11 years her BMI $= 27.3$, below the 99.6[th] centile, plotted on the WHO/UK 1990 female BMI charts. Waist:height ratio $- 66/136 = 0.48$, no health risks indicated.

Continuing the Management Pathway

For weight management in CYP, the pathway for treatment has typically stopped at family lifestyle management. Bariatric surgery for adolescents has been an option that has not always been fully embraced but should have a place in a comprehensive pathway for adolescents, particularly those with extreme obesity. The use of new generation pharmacology for CYP is really only beginning to be seen in practice and has an interesting future. These newer approaches are discussed below.

Both of these sections have been included in this chapter to give a rounded overview of the options available for all CYP living with obesity. It should be noted that in most regions these options will only be available for those young people living with severe obesity.

Bariatric Surgery

The British Obesity and Metabolic Surgery Society (BOMSS) describes bariatric and metabolic surgery as *'a treatment option for people with severe obesity. Bariatric surgery should be seen as part of a comprehensive approach, which includes lifestyle management'* (Bariatric and Metabolic Surgery (`bomss.org`)).

While there are a number of surgical bariatric procedures, currently in the UK (and across the world) the gastric bypass and the sleeve gastrectomy are the most common. Bariatric surgery, also called metabolic surgery, was once considered to induce significant weight loss due to the restriction of energy intake from food combined with a malabsorption of energy along with other nutrients. However, it is now recognised that the surgery alters the state of communication in the gut-brain axis, which includes hormones and the gut microbial flora. These changes appear to alter the signalling relating to satiety and hunger passing between the brain and gut [18, 19].

The AAP 2023 guidelines recommend that bariatric surgery has a role in treatment of paediatric obesity when it is part of a comprehensive package of care and is carried out by a team experienced in paediatric bariatric surgery [3]. While the NICE 2023 guidelines concur with this, they state that bariatric surgery should only be considered *'in exceptional circumstances'* and when a young person has *'achieved or nearly achieved physiological maturity'* [2].

The AAP notes that the laparoscopic Roux-en-Y gastric bypass and the vertical sleeve gastrectomy are the most commonly performed in this age group [3]. As with adults being considered for bariatric surgery, it is important to ensure comprehensive pre-surgery assessments are carried out including a risk-benefit analysis, specialist assessment for eating disorders and psychological assessment [2]. Additionally, post-surgery follow-up by a multi-disciplinary team is equally important [20].

A Cochrane Library review from 2015 looked for RCTs of surgical interventions for treating CYP, aged less than 18 years and living with obesity, where there had been a minimum of 6 months follow-up [21]. Only one study met their inclusion criteria. This study had been undertaken in Australia and included a total of 50 young people who had been randomised in a group receiving a laparoscopic adjustable gastric band compared to a lifestyle usual care group, with follow-up at 24 months [22]. It is important to note that the Cochrane reviewers, using the Grading of Recommendations Assessment, Development and Evaluation (GRADE) framework (What is GRADE?|BMJ Best Practice), considered the evidence quality to be low.

At two years, the study had reported a mean change in weight among its subjects of −34.6 kg (CI 30.2–39) in the intervention group compared to −3.0 kg (CI 2.1–8.1) in the usual care group. This 2015 Cochrane review concluded that there was insufficient good quality evidence to make an informed recommendation [21]. A 2022 update of the same Cochrane review found no further evidence, i.e. no new RCTs that met the review's criteria. They came to the same conclusion that there was insufficient good quality evidence [23].

While there may be limited good quality RCTs, bariatric surgery as a pathway option for young people living with severe and extreme obesity is an important option for teams to consider and explore.

Pharmacology

While some pharmacology has been approved and used with young people, such as Orlistat typically from age 12 [24], the first part of this section intends to concentrate on the next generation of anti-obesity medications. These medications have been developed and approved for use in for adults, and some countries are starting to look to approving them for use with CYP, again typically from age 12 years and older.

The developmental starting point for these next-generation medications were the hormones affecting the gut-brain axis. One such gut hormone is Glucagon-like peptide 1 (GLP-1), which is released naturally by the body upon eating. It is known to slow down gastric emptying as well as being part of the gut-brain dialogue on satiety by decreasing hunger signals. It has successfully been used in the management of type 2 diabetes [25] and has been found to be successful in inducing weight loss in adults [26, 27]. RCT studies of lifestyle interventions and GLP-1s versus placebo in adolescents, aged 12–18 years, are also showing greater weight loss for the GLP-1 group [28, 29].

GLP-1s tend to be administered by injection, some daily others weekly, which may be off-putting for some adolescents. Oral GLP-1s are certainly being developed and considered for weight loss in adults [30] and will likely be approved and available to adolescents in the future. It is important to consider and explain the reported and possible side effects of these drugs, which include nausea, vomiting and diarrhoea. It is essential that the use of medication for weight loss management in young people includes frequent and regular follow-ups and should only be used within the support of a multi-disciplinary team.

The other type of next-generation anti-obesity medications are those developed to combat monogenetic causes of obesity [31], such as leptin deficiency and defects in the MC4R pathway [32]. The use of these medications is extremely specialised as, for example, in the UK they are only licensed for prescription by the lead of GOOS (Home – Genetics of Obesity Study (goos.org.uk)). With the low numbers of CYP reported with these monogenetic causes for the obesity, these will be a niche but important tool for any service to consider.

WHAT DOES THIS MEAN IN PRACTICE?

- A childhood weight management service can be delivered by a multi-disciplinary team or a uni-profession with links to other services.
- Programmes need to incorporate necessary lifestyle changes while being person-centred and using behavioural change tools.
- The involvement of the family and the importance of parent (adult) role modelling should be emphasised.
- Bariatric and metabolic surgery should be part of a childhood weight management pathway, following the local/national guidance on eligibility.
- New generation pharmacology is a useful addition for clinicians to consider in childhood weight management services.

References

1 Stewart, L. (2008). Personal communication: parent.
2 NICE (2023). Obesity: identification, assessment and management. https://www.nice.org.uk/guidance/cg189 (accessed 1 June 2024).
3 Hampl, S.E., Hassink, S.G., Skinner, A.C. et al. (2023). Clinical practice guideline for the evaluation and treatment of children and adolescents with obesity. *Pediatrics* 151: e2022060640. https://doi.org/10.1542/peds.2022-060640.
4 NHS Health Scotland (2019). standards-for-the-delivery-of-tier-2-and-tier-3-weight-management-services-for-children-and-young-people-in-scotland-english-oct2019.pdf (healthscotland.scot) (accessed 29 March 2024).
5 Hayes, J., Altman, M., Coppock, J. et al. (2015). Recent updates on the efficacy of group based treatments for pediatric obesity. *Curr. Cardiovasc. Risk Rep.* 9: 2–17. https://doi.org/10.1007/s12170-015-0443-8.
6 Gray, L.A., Hernandez Alava, M., Kelly, M.P. et al. (2018). Family lifestyle dynamics and childhood obesity: evidence from the millennium cohort study. *BMC Public Health* 18: 1–15. https://doi.org/10.1186/s12889-018-5398-5.
7 Golan, M. (2006). Parents as agents of change in childhood obesity – from research to practice. *Int. J. Pediatr. Obes.* 1: 66–76. https://doi.org/10.1080/17477160600644272.
8 Loveman, E., Re, J., Robertson, W. et al. (2015). Parent-only interventions for childhood overweight or obesity in children aged 5 to 11 years. *Cochrane Database Syst. Rev.* 1–205. https://doi.org/10.1002/14651858.CD012008.
9 Stewart, L., Houghton, J., Hughes, A.R. et al. (2005). Dietetic management of pediatric overweight: development and description of a practical and evidence-based behavioral approach. *J. Am. Diet. Assoc.* 105: 1810–1815. https://doi.org/10.1016/j.jada.2005.08.006.

10 Sacher, P.M., Kolotourou, M., Chadwick, P.M. et al. (2010). Randomized controlled trial of the MEND program: a family-based community intervention for childhood obesty. *Obesity* 18: S62–S68: https://doi.org/10.1038/oby.2009.433.

11 Martin, L., Greci, S., NHS Health Scotland (2019). Summary of highly processed evidence on components of effective weight management interventions for children and young people. http://www.healthscotland.scot/media/2657/summary-of-evidence-for-effective-weight-management-interventions.pdf (accessed 1 June 2024).

12 Ho, M., Garnett, S.P., Baur, L. et al. (2012). Effectiveness of lifestyle interventions in child obesity: systematic review with meta-analysis. *Pediatrics* 130:https://doi.org/10.1542/peds.2012-1176.

13 Stewart, L., Chapple, J., Hughes, A.R. et al. (2008). The use of behavioural change techniques in the treatment of paediatric obesity: qualitative evaluation of parental perspectives on treatment. *J. Hum. Nutr. Diet.* 21: 464–473. https://doi.org/10.1111/j.1365-277X.2008.00888.x.

14 Baur, L.A. (2015). Early clinical interventions and outcomes. In: *Early Years Nutrition and Healthy Weight* (ed. L. Stewart and J. Thompson), 100–111. Wiley.

15 Stewart, L. (2020). Obesity. In: *Clinical Paediatric Dietetics*, 5e (ed. V. Shaw). Wiley, p. 472.

16 Stewart, L. and Easter, S. (2021). BDA's obesity specialist group. British dietetic association's obesity specialist group dietetic obesity management interventions in children and young people: review & clinical application. *J. Hum. Nutr. Diet.* 34: 224–232. https://doi.org/10.1111/jhn.12834.

17 BDA (2016). Model and process for nutrition and dietetic practice. 2021-BDA-Model-and-Process-for-Nutrition-and-Dietetic-Practice.pdf (accessed 29 March 2024).

18 Pucci, A. and Batterham, R.L. (2020). Endocrinology of the gut and the regulation of body weight and metabolism. In: *Endotext* (ed. K.R. Feingold, B. Anawalt, M.R. Blackman, et al.). South Dartmouth (MA): Endotext.org http://www.ncbi.nlm.nih.gov/pubmed/32352695.

19 Dimitriadis, G.K., Randeva, M.S., and Miras, A.D. (2017). Potential hormone mechanisms of bariatric surgery. *Curr. Obes. Rep.* 6: 253–265. https://doi.org/10.1007/s13679-017-0276-5.

20 Elhag, W. and El Ansari, W. (2022). Multiple nutritional deficiencies among adolescents undergoing bariatric surgery: who is at risk? *Surg. Obes. Relat. Dis.* 18: 413–424. https://doi.org/10.1016/j.soard.2021.10.024.

21 Ells, L.J., Mead, E., Atkinson, G. et al. (2015). Surgery for the treatment of obesity in children and adolescents. *Cochrane Database Syst. Rev.* https://doi.org/10.1002/14651858.CD011740.

22 O'Brien, P.E., Sawyer, S.M., Laurie, C. et al. (2010). Laparoscopic adjustable gastric banding in severely obese adolescents: a randomized trial. *JAMA* 303: 519–526. https://doi.org/10.1001/jama.2010.81.

23 Torbahn, G., Brauchmann, J., Axon, E. et al. (2022). Surgery for the treatment of obesity in children and adolescents. *Cochrane Database Syst. Rev.* https://doi.org/10.1002/14651858.CD011740.pub2.

24 Chanoine, J.-P., Hampl, S., Jensen, C. et al. (2005). Effect of orlistat on weight and body composition in obese adolescents. *JAMA* 293: 2873. https://doi.org/10.1001/jama.293.23.2873.

25 Scheen, A.J. (2007). Glucagon-like peptide-1 (GLP-1), new target for the treatment of type 2 diabetes. *Rev. Med. Liege* 62: 217–221.

26 Vilsbøll, T., Christensen, M., Junker, A.E. et al. (2012). Effects of glucagon-like peptide-1 receptor agonists on weight loss: systematic review and meta-analyses of randomised controlled trials. *BMJ* 344: 1–11. https://doi.org/10.1136/bmj.d7771.

27 Singh, G., Krauthamer, M., and Bjalme-Evans, M. (2022). Wegovy (semaglutide): a new weight loss drug for chronic weight management. *J. Investig. Med.* 70: 5–13. https://doi.org/10.1136/jim-2021-001952.

28 Kelly, A.S., Auerbach, P., Barrientos-Perez, M. et al. (2020). A randomized, controlled trial of liraglutide for adolescents with obesity. *N. Engl. J. Med.* 382: 2117–2128. https://doi.org/10.1056/nejmoa1916038.

29 Weghuber, D., Barrett, T., Barrientos-Pérez, M. et al. (2022). Once-weekly semaglutide in adolescents with obesity. *N. Engl. J. Med.* 387: 2245–2257. https://doi.org/10.1056/nejmoa2208601.

30 Wharton, S., Blevins, T., Connery, L. et al. (2023). Daily oral GLP-1 receptor agonist orforglipron for adults with obesity. *N. Engl. J. Med.* 389: 877–888. https://doi.org/10.1056/NEJMoa2302392.

31 Van Der Klaauw, A.A. and Farooqi, I.S. (2015). The hunger genes: pathways to obesity. *Cell* 161: 119–132. https://doi.org/10.1016/j.cell.2015.03.008.

32 Clément, K., van den Akker, E., Argente, J. et al. (2020). Efficacy and safety of setmelanotide, an MC4R agonist, in individuals with severe obesity due to LEPR or POMC deficiency: single-arm, open-label, multicentre, phase 3 trials. *Lancet Diabetes Endocrinol.* 8: 960–970. https://doi.org/10.1016/S2213-8587(20)30364-8.

12 Adolescent Weight Management
The Factors for Clinicians to Be Aware

Clare Q Neilson

'and with GCSEs and mocks for people who have other issues to deal with like weight … it's easy to give up and say I can't do it when I compare myself to other people'. [1]

Introduction

While obesity is a multifactorial disease, this chapter will focus on the challenges faced by adolescents living in an obesogenic environment while simultaneously navigating the physiological and neurological development which they are undergoing. In 2016, 18% of the worldwide adolescent population (324 million individuals) were living with overweight or obesity; this figure represented an increase of 120% from 1900 [2]. Strikingly, in Europe 1:4 live with overweight or obesity [3].

The broad themes to be explored here are the influence of **developmental factors** (parenting style, emotional eating /interpersonal conflict, neurodevelopment, neurodiversity, hormonal changes, diversity and the impact of adverse childhood experiences), **environmental factors** (including home environment and cultural influences) and the role of **lifestyle** (sleep, physical activity and pregnancy) on adolescent eating habits. The term adolescence will be used exclusively throughout this chapter to refer to those young people who are in the phase of transition from childhood into adulthood. This is a stage in life where the young person has limited control; they have limited autonomy, except for their self-governance of disposable income and food preferences. Adolescents are also at the 'mercy' of and under the influence of social media while also being highly susceptible to advertising [4].

Child and Adolescent Obesity: A Practical Approach to Clinical Weight Management,
First Edition. Edited by Laura Stewart.
© 2024 John Wiley & Sons Ltd. Published 2024 by John Wiley & Sons Ltd.

In adolescence, the impact of some early life experiences become evident and the adverse consequences that these experiences have had become apparent. Habits and behaviours arising from previous experiences, learning environments and genetic programming rise to prominence.

> Clinically, what do we need to be aware of to be of greatest benefit to the young person we are working with?

Parental Role

Parents influence the weight status of young people in several ways. They provide, they model and they influence the young person's environment. Parental weight status remains a reliable predictor of a CYP's weight and the style of parenting experiences which are provided is influential on a CYP's weight status [5]. The genetic contribution made by parents is only part of the picture, and the role of parental behaviour is central to the development of the young adult. For the young adults, the eating environment they have experienced shapes their future behaviour and influences their own parenting style for the future generation.

Julie was a 20-year-old first time mother who was adopted at an early age. Her experience of childhood was stressful and has resulted in her being anxious about the experience of being a mother. She lacked positive role models; her individual experiences of childhood were mixed. Her first child, Rowan, was born 17 years ago and the magnitude of motherhood was overwhelming for her. Julie attempted to parent in a way which came intuitively, although this was affected by spells of anxiety and low mood at points in Rowan's life. Rowan recalls that Julie was 'keen to be a friend' suggesting that even from a young age Rowan could sense their mother's informal approach to her parental role.

Parenting **style** is categorised into four domains, each with varying levels of warmth and responsiveness compared against levels of control and demandingness, from authoritative (high warmth, high control), authoritarian (low warmth, high control), indulgent (high warmth, low control), to uninvolved (low warmth, low control) [6, 7], for greater discussion on parenting style, see Chapter 10. The **quality** of parenting has been assessed using a three 7-point scales: emotional support, respect for the child's autonomy and hostility [8]. The **quality** of parenting has been implicated in subsequent adolescent eating behaviour and linked to the emergence of emotional eating in adolescents who have experienced poorer quality parenting, so clinically a clear developmental history is essential for implementation of any treatment plan [8].

Parenting style, feeding style and food-parenting practices have been extensively investigated, and it is accepted that parenting style refers to the emotional reciprocity within the parent–child relationship [5]. Parental feeding style and food-parenting practice have been shown to be associated with the development of diet-related self-regulatory behaviour and the concept of **'food parenting'** has been explored in the various developmental stages. With reference to adolescence, Balantekin et al. combine the parenting style constructs with feeding practices. They have highlighted the value of a parenting style with monitoring, boundary setting while modelling and praise are also present showing that this leads to self-determination where health and related behaviours are positive – Figure 12.1 shows the continuum at each stage of development [5].

Following Rowan's birth Julie's mood deteriorated, and she was soon diagnosed with postnatal depression. Parenting Rowan was challenging. Over time Julie recovered, although she continued to utilise food as a source of comfort. It became evident that Julie's parenting style was indulgent: emotionally she was attuned to her child's needs but she did not have boundaries or routines in place for Rowan. Consequently, from an early age they eat when and where they wanted and what they wanted. However, due to changes in Julie's mental health, there could be times when food was scarce within the house and Rowan recalls this.

Interpersonal Conflict Leading to Emotional Eating

The adolescent years are notorious for being a time of strife. This can be evident in the domestic setting, among peer groups and ultimately in any interpersonal interactions. There are many factors that contribute to this, and several are elaborated upon here including hormone changes and behaviours; both those modelled by others, either within or outwith the home, and those arising from experiential learning during the formative years. We know that conflict alone does not lead to weight change, but the emotional impact of conflict can [9]. The behavioural response to emotional distress can be learned or modelled and often comfort eating results as a method of self-soothing. The ability to regulate

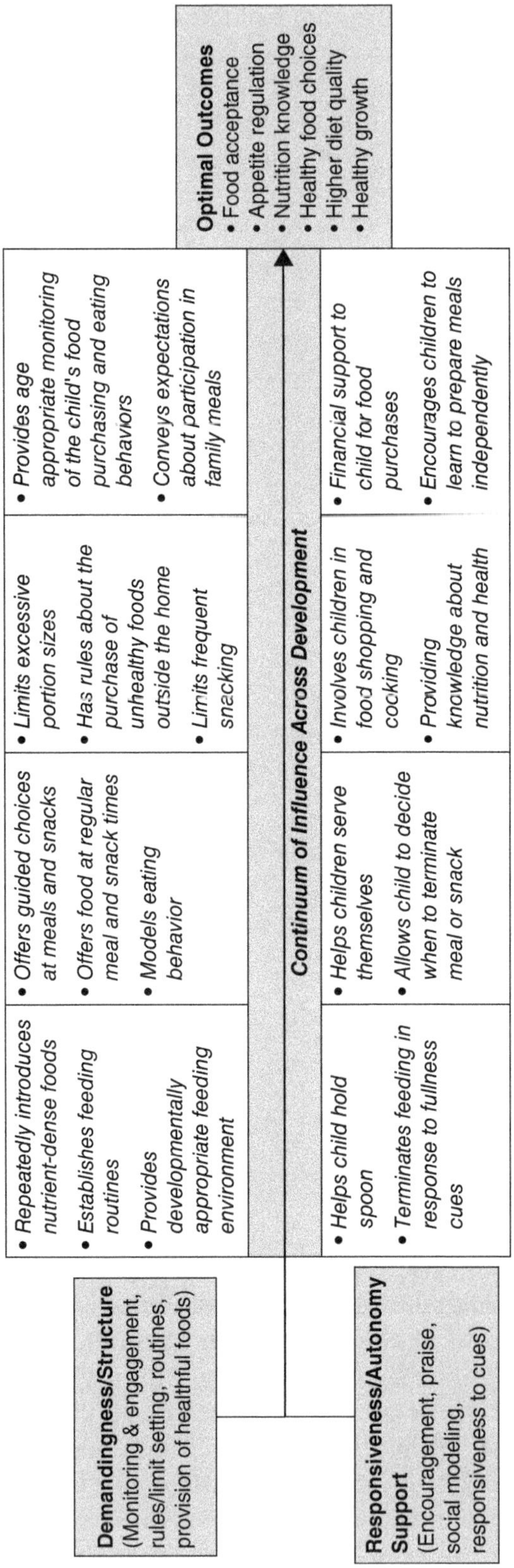

Demandingness/Structure
(Monitoring & engagement, rules/limit setting, routines, provision of healthful foods)

	Infancy	Early Childhood	Middle Childhood	Adolescence
	• Repeatedly introduces nutrient-dense foods • Establishes feeding routines • Provides developmentally appropriate feeding environment	• Offers guided choices at meals and snacks • Offers food at regular meal and snack times • Models eating behavior	• Limits excessive portion sizes • Has rules about the purchase of unhealthy foods outside the home • Limits frequent snacking	• Provides age appropriate monitoring of the child's food purchasing and eating behaviors • Conveys expectations about participation in family meals

Continuum of Influence Across Development →

Responsiveness/Autonomy Support
(Encouragement, praise, social modeling, responsiveness to cues)

	Infancy	Early Childhood	Middle Childhood	Adolescence
	• Helps child hold spoon • Terminates feeding in response to fullness cues	• Helps children serve themselves • Allows child to decide when to terminate meal or snack	• Involves children in food shopping and cooking • Providing knowledge about nutrition and health	• Financial support to child for food purchases • Encourages children to learn to prepare meals independently

Optimal Outcomes
- Food acceptance
- Appetite regulation
- Nutrition knowledge
- Healthy food choices
- Higher diet quality
- Healthy growth

Figure 12.1 Illustrating the continuum at each stage of development.

Source: Reproduced from Balantekin et al. [5]/with permission of John Wiley & Sons.

emotional states can fail to develop due to early life experiences, therefore emotional eating (EE) is linked to an individual's attempt to emotional self-regulation [10]. EE is conceptualised as *eating behaviour which serves as a coping mechanism in response to stress or negative feelings* and EE is linked to increased risk of binge eating behaviour, eating when hunger is not present and obesity risk. The association between EE and binge-eating behaviours in adolescence has been investigated and in particular the intergenerational transmission pathways associated with emotional feeding and adolescent binge-eating behaviour [11]. The requirement for clinicians working with adolescents to take EE into account when delivering treatment is essential [12].

Shriver et al. have explored 138, 17-year-olds' EE and its association with emotion regulation in childhood, adolescent weight status, body image and emotional eating. They concluded that interdisciplinary interventions focused on cognitive behavioural factors in addition to dietetic and physical activity are required to address EE in adolescence because it arises from emotional dysregulation, weight status and negative body image [13]. Maternal EE and mental health difficulties have been found to link with increased weight status. It is interesting to consider this in relation to the effects of parental modelling of behaviours and poorer quality parenting, which has also been associated with suppression of emotions, difficulty identifying emotions and greater levels of EE in adolescence [8, 14].

As an adolescent, Rowan seeks solace in school where they immerse themselves in extra-curricular activities and academic work. Life at home is not easy. Rowan now has three siblings who are in need of physical and emotional care. Rowan's relationship with Julie is strained due to Julie's heavy drinking and her prolonged spells of absence from the home. Rowan has mixed emotions towards Julie: a desire to be supported and nurtured by a mother but also an awareness of the need to support and nurture the siblings and Julie. Time spent with mum usually involves an argument or hostile silence. Rowan describes 'eating their feelings' and over-eating and binging in an attempt to feeling 'something', even if that is pain or discomfort.

Neurodevelopment

When we are engaging with adolescents in weight-related work, we must be aware of the role neurological factors play in their presentations, and while the specifics of neurobiology and neurophysiology along with neuropsychology are out with the scope of this chapter, we must acknowledge the role of the brain in appetite regulation and mood. The environment, genetics and hormonal factors all interact with complex neurophysiological processes to regulate human eating, and obesity is indicative of a breakdown in the appetite-communication system [15].

Neurodiversity

By virtue of being human we are heterogeneous and therefore diversity of attributes enhances and enriches us and the communities in which we live. However, those living with neurodiverse conditions can be poorly understood by others. Health-related behaviours, including eating, are impacted upon for people with neurodiverse conditions in particular autistic spectrum disorder (ASD) and attention-deficit hyperactivity disorder (ADHD). Please refer to Chapter 14 for more information specifically on Children living with Additional Support Needs, here we are thinking about the adolescent living with neurodiversity.

As referred to previously, an individual's neurodevelopment impacts upon their eating behaviour and this can be further compounded by neurodiversity. Some of the coping strategies or self-soothing behaviours employed can directly and indirectly lead to increased weight status. In a recent meta-analysis of the prevalence of adolescents living with ADHD, it was found that 20.9% were living with overweight and 14.4% living with obesity, and for those living with ASD it was found that 19.8% were living with overweight and 21.8% living with obesity [16]. It may seem paradoxical to consider ADHD as co-existing with obesity, *'these people are constantly on the go, how is it possible for them to have a higher weight status than their non-neurodiverse peers?'*, maybe a view held. However, there is increasing evidence to suggest that there is a relationship [17, 18] although this view is not universally accepted [19].

The prevalence of adolescents with ASD is increasing, and they are at greater risk of obesity than their peers without ASD [20]. Nor et al. report that these findings hold internationally, with similar findings in Malaysian adolescents [21]. Cowling et al. report on improvements which could be made within the UK to the routine gathering of clinical data in order to improve clinical care to adolescents with neurodevelopmental conditions and obesity [22]. Sammels et al. reiterate the finding that few European studies have established an association between obesity prevalence in adolescents with and without ASD, the data that does exist predominately hails from North America [23].

No formal diagnosis has even been given to Rowan, but they have several traits associated with ASD. Their preference for solitary pursuits and desire to socialise via computer-based interactions and 'gaming' are some of the examples of this. Rowan has a younger sibling who has a diagnosis of ASD and acknowledges many similarities between them, especially associated with a 'lack of connectedness'. A formal diagnosis is not something Rowan seeks, preferring to develop an idiographic understanding of their behaviours and the precipitants and perpetuates of these: those factors which underpin and cause personal actions in addition to the factors which maintain these behaviours.

Hormones

Adolescence is a time in life when the body is undergoing extensive change, development and growth. When we are working clinically with adolescents living with increased weight status, we must remember that their age-related hormonal changes will also be impacting on their presentation. Little is understood of the interaction of puberty on the production of appetite-related hormones but Patel et al. concluded that the production of these hormones is correlated during pubertal development with sex and weight status [24]. What this suggests is that we must be alert to the stage of development, gender and self-perceptions of appetite.

A person's gender, stage of puberty, weight status and mental health must be considered when a weight loss intervention is being proposed. During adolescence, observations of behaviour indicate that mental health negatively correlates with weight status [25]. In addition, links between estrogen and progesterone levels have been found to influence emotional eating among menstruating females [26].

The mental health of the individual has an impact upon their appetite and eating behaviour, and the reciprocal association between depression and obesity has been established for adults [27, 28]. Whether or not the same reciprocal relationship exists for adolescents is less clear, and there would appear to be cultural influences on this [29]. A large meta-analysis involving 51,272 young people Quek et al. identified that adolescents with obesity were at increased risk of depression with female and non-Western individuals at greatest risk [30].

Polycystic ovarian syndrome (PCOS) is caused by a hormonal imbalance characterised by increased weight status and reproductive implications and although the presence of PCOS does not become apparent clinically until adolescence, it is believed that evidence of its existence can be seen at a much younger age [31]. The co-existence of

PCOS and psychological distress has been investigated and the increased risk of obesity, PCOS, binge eating and psychological distress have been explored [32]. Therefore, when working with adolescent females for whom weight is problematic, we must be alert to the potential presence of PCOS in a client and its relationship to their eating behaviour.

Rowan's self-reports that at age 5 their weight status was greater than their peers and by the time of puberty this was more apparent, and food served as a source of distraction and comfort. When Rowan's mood was low, food was a companion. We also know that Rowan has a maternal predisposition to anxiety and depression, their mother having had episodes of each during her lifetime and this genetic inheritance may be evident during the hormonal upheaval of puberty for Rowan.

Weight Stigma

Stigma can be detrimental to the formation of self-identity which is underway during adolescence and those who are or self-identify as being, overweight are at greater risk of stigmatisation. Stigmatisation of people with obesity is prevalent and extremely harmful. It can be seen on social media, playgrounds and workplaces and it can impact on mental health, psychological well-being, engagement in activities of daily living, on an adolescent's quality of life and ultimately their future. The impact of stigma can be life-long and the effects can be experienced indefinitely. Some in society continue to hold a misplaced belief that creating stigma through teasing, shame or embarrassment can be motivators of change, prompting people to lose weight. Far from promoting health behaviour changes [33], this approach contributes to binge eating, decreased physical activity, social isolation and weight gain compounding their unhealthy weight status. This then perpetuates the cycle of avoidance and resistance to health behaviour change. Hooper et al. identified that weight stigma correlated with a greater number of unhealthy behaviours, including screen-time, intensity of physical activity and fast food consumption [34].

Throughout school, Rowan has experienced bullying in various forms and to varying degrees, from teasing about being a geek, to emotional bullying about their weight status and there have been incidents of physical violence: being tripped up in the corridor, having their belongings scattered around the playground and being mocked with animal noises being chanted as they collected them. Rowan is only too familiar with overt and covert weight stigma.

Rowan does not feel connected to others, they do not feel as though they belong, and this is compounded by being overweight and the years of teasing and name calling they have experienced.

Body image dissatisfaction presents in adolescence and impacts on mood, self-esteem, eating behaviour, weight stigma and teasing. Wang et al. found almost 95% of the 1455 sample had body image dissatisfaction from adolescence and this was associated with increased weight status [35].

Sexual and Gender Diversity

If gender identity is an individual's personal understanding of their true gender, then gender diversity is the acknowledgement and respect that there are many ways to identify other than the binary male and female forms, for those whose personal understanding of their true gender is diverse. Services must ensure inclusivity of all clients and the use of preferred names and pronouns for gender diverse people and the use of gender-neutral language are all part of inclusivity [36–38].

Diversity, of either sexuality or gender identity, can be experienced during adolescence and for a variety of reasons, including weigh-based victimisation, weight stigma, self-esteem, body dissatisfaction and mood, it can be associated with increased weight status [39–41]. Sexual and gender diversity has been linked with increased weight status [42]. Himmelstein et al. have investigated weight-based victimisation, eating behaviour and health behaviours within this population. It was found that this type of victimisation and stigma may contribute to unhelpful eating and ultimately obesity [41]. Gender diverse adolescents have been found to be at increased risk of having obesity and to experience weight or size-related victimisation compared to cisgender peers [43].

Mental well-being in gender diverse adolescents can be impacted upon and adversely affect social functioning and emotional well-being [44], which can in turn trigger EE and the emotional dysregulation discussed previously and may or may not produce an increase in weight status.

Clinicians working with gender diverse adolescents must be aware who they are and the different ways this can influence their weight status.

Sleep

Sleep hygiene has been covered in Chapter 5, but it continues to be as important for adolescents. Researchers distinguish between the length of sleep – sleep duration and the regularity of sleep – the timing of sleep, and it has been found that variations in both the amount and the regularity of sleep are associated with obesity [45] and also increased food intake, poor diet quality and increased weight status [46]. Furthermore, the relationship between sleep (poor quality and quantity), food cravings and obesity have again underlined the role of sleep in adolescents' dietary behaviour [47]. Some argue that it is duration of sleep which is associated with adolescent obesity [48, 49].

A potential relationship between PCOS, the condition arising from a hormonal imbalance, and sleep disturbance has been explored, and the need for the assessment of sleep to be core component of adolescents with PCOS and obesity has been highlighted [50].

Physical Activity

The role of physical activity, as with sleep, has been explored in a previous chapter, but it is worth reminding clinicians of the relevance of physical activity to adolescents. All-too-often adolescents do not have a positive relationship with physical activity, and this is especially the case for females [51, 52]. Therefore, in relation to maintaining a healthy weight status, this is challenging because low levels of physical activity and high levels of sedentary behaviour correlate with increased weight status [53]. We also know of the mental health benefits of physical activity and the negative impact of sedentary behaviour on mental health [54].

Rowan reports having had problems with sleep, both a difficulty getting off to sleep and the quality of sleep. The draw of gaming and the prospect of socialising with 'invisible' friends around the world often overshadows the need for sleep. Rowan acknowledges that while 'burning the midnight oil', they are often consuming snacks.

Lack of self-esteem, poor body image and living in a larger body are all reasons Rowan gives for avoiding physical activity in school.

Pregnancy

Adolescence is a time of increasing independence and sexual experimentation often occurs, which can result in teenage pregnancy and consequently clinicians working with adolescents to manage their weight status need to be aware of the risks associated with pregnancy, weight status and maternal and infant outcomes. The WHO reported that each year 12 million girls aged 15–19 give birth, although the teenage birth rate is decreasing in Western countries [55]. Pregnancy and childbirth during adolescence is more prevalent among those with less social advantage across Europe [56]. For decades, international researchers have been reporting on the health risks to women and their babies [57] and the impact of increased weight status correlates with various pregnancy outcomes [58]. Therefore, the clinical relevance of this is that the core principles of healthy eating prevail and the effects of parenting style, food-parenting, stigma, maternal mental health and trauma also all need to be assessed and the impact these have upon two generations: the maternal adolescent and the infant; and the next generation [59].

Social Injustice

Practitioners must remain alert to the social circumstances, ethnicity, faith, cultural background and race of the people they work. We must remember that every family-unit has its own culture, its own routines and traditions, and we must be cognisant of this when working in a person-centred way. The socioeconomic gradient of obesity has been documented and describes the inverse relationship that exists between obesity and low SES. In high-income countries lower SES has long been linked with an increased risk of higher weight status [60].

In Scotland, between 1998 and 2014, rates of obesity increased for the most disadvantaged 40% of 2- to 15-year-olds, while the prevalence of obesity remained stable for those in the most advantaged areas [61] with similar findings in Ireland [62]. In a longitudinal UK-based study [63] reporting on 15996, 3- to 14-year-olds, risks of increased weight status by ethnicity during adolescence and reported that higher SES may not always correlate with healthier weight status.

Furthermore, lower SES and health inequalities are highly correlated with adverse childhood experiences, which in turn have been found to precipitate overweight and obesity amongst young people. There are many consequences of low SES which have been investigated among adolescents, including poorer educational achievement, and poorer mental and physical health outcomes [64–66].

Adverse Childhood Events

The experience of adversity in early life has been shown to have a dose-related relationship with adverse developmental and psychological outcomes [67]. Although there is not a definitive list of ACEs, it is accepted that experiences in early life that are not considered to be typical to childhood and exceed the coping resources of the average child should be considered within this category. These experiences include, but are not limited to, all forms of violence and threats to safety arising from physical, sexual, and emotional abuse and neglect, including bullying, domestic violence, crime, death and loss of a parent, e.g. parental incapacitation and absence. Felitti and colleagues established the causal link between abuse – physical, sexual, or emotional – domestic disharmony and the impact on health-related behaviour and disease in adulthood [68]. Our understanding of the wider impacts on health has developed, and it is appreciated that ACEs can have a direct consequence upon weight status [65, 69]. Perhaps unsurprisingly, EE has been found to be prevalent among those who have experienced ACEs [70].

Although it is not being suggested that all adolescents living with obesity have experienced multiple ACEs [64], many studies have found a relationship between experience of ACEs and obesity [71, 72]. There is evidence to support the belief that exposure to an increased number of ACEs leads to incremental increase in weight status [73].

Based on all that is known about the negative impact ACEs have upon young people, clinicians would be negligent if they failed to explore this further with their clients. At a national level, the UK government and providers of healthcare have set out expectations for society to have an increased awareness of trauma-related experiences and the subsequent effects including the development of trauma informed practice [74]. Beyond the UK, a number of other countries have also taken steps to address the impact of trauma on weight gain [75–77].

Additional Factors for Clinical Consideration

Adolescence is characterised by increasing independence in decision-making with the reduction of parental influence and increased influence of peers and social media, which influence eating behaviours both directly and indirectly. Adolescents may also have paid employment and therefore access to disposable income, and the choices they make about how to spend their money can have an adverse impact on their weight status. Social opportunities also emerge, and these coupled with financial means can contribute to the consumption of alcohol, such as the highly calorific alcoho-pops which are marketed at adolescents.

In clinic, when working with adolescents we must continue to assess their habits, behaviours, and routines just as we do with all of our clients irrespective of their age.

Rowan experienced multiple ACES beginning in infancy when Julie had difficulty bonding with Rowan, resulting in emotional distance between mother and child and the infant could have experienced this as emotional neglect.

Rowan experienced the separation of their parents when aged 5-years-old and then aged 6 Rowan recalls the class teacher sharing a newspaper article which detailed the conviction and incarceration of their father. Julie moved her new partner into their home, and he remained for six years – these were not happy times for Rowan. They have disclosed that an incident of sexual assault occurred when Rowan was 12-years-old, perpetrated by 'a friend' of Julie's partner. Rowan never felt able to tell Julie as they do not think they would be believed. There was further evidence of emotional neglect when Rowan's siblings were born, and they became the focus of Julie's attention. Rowan experienced and witnessed acts of physical threats and violence at the hands of Julie's partner – on one occasion Rowan recalls being hit with an iron and the imprint of the hot metal being left on their skin. Julie and Rowan's step-father spent many evenings out drinking in the local bar, leaving Rowan to care for the three siblings. The family experienced significant financial hardship and as they got older Rowan took on more of the parental roles with their siblings – cooking, cleaning, and washing and ironing clothes for them.

Julie has a new partner, but now aged 18 Rowan has left the family home although they have immense feelings of guilt at leaving their siblings. Rowan's view is that the siblings have been 'abandoned' and Rowan identifies similar feelings when their biological father left their life. When at school, Rowan loved to read, to listen to and to play music – these passions Rowan describes as having been 'saviours'. School orchestras and English classes were 'safe places'. Rowan is now at university studying English with no support, emotional or financial, from Julie. They are happy, they say, except with how they look and their weight. At age 18 years and 1 month, Rowan weighs 180.351 kg (their height is 160.4 cm, giving them a BMI of 71.6).

Rowan wants to 'lose weight', but, as we know, it is not as simple as that. There are many factors to be addressed before weight status will change.

Making Sense of this Clinically

The various influences on adolescent weight status discussed in this chapter should be explored during the assessment and will in turn have a bearing on the interventions adopted. It can be helpful to consider the approach taken by psychologists using a process referred to as 'formulation' [78, 79]. A formulation involves utilising the biopsychosocial information obtained at the assessment to create a shared understanding of the client's reasons for presenting for treatment. The **presenting difficulty** is identified and in the context of this chapter, that is weight status or 'why someone has developed the relationship with food that they have'. The various **predisposing factors** which include genetic, neonatal and historical aspects of an individual which are relevant to the development of increased weight status are identified. Consideration is then given to those factors which are considered to have contributed to the individual's weight and ultimately their relationship with food: the **precipitating factors** and those that are believed to be maintaining the presenting difficulty (the **perpetuating factors**) are identified. It is also important to highlight the elements that are seen as protective, these **protective factors** are what help to buffer the client from day-to-day emotional and situational challenges.

WHAT DOES THIS MEAN IN PRACTICE?

When working clinically with adolescents, clinicians need to make an informal assessment of the person's developmental and environmental experiences: their early life experiences and emotional attachments to significant caregivers as well as the style of parenting they experienced. An understanding of how the individual manages emotional distress provides information about the presence or not of emotional eating. Emotional eating can lead to the creation of weight stigma which in turn can have a causal relationship with poor sleep habits, disengagement from physical activity increase in sedentary behaviour. Hormonal changes and the neurodevelopment that occurs during adolescence must also be taken into account. Social injustice and being different can play a significant role in the development of negative weight-related behaviour and therefore must be explored by practitioners. ACEs impact on the emotional development, the environmental situation and lifestyle choices made by adolescents.

References

1 Rigby, E., McKoewn, R., and Wortley, L. (2022). The experiences of young people and their families living with excess weight: themes from engagement work. https://ayph.org.uk/wp-content/uploads/2022/04/CEW-Themes-from-engagement-work.pdf (accessed 18 February 2023).

2 Azzopardi, P.S., Hearps, S.J.C., Francis, K.L. et al. (2019). Progress in adolescent health and wellbeing: tracking 12 headline indicators for 195 countries and territories, 1990–2016. *Lancet (London, England)* 393: 1101–1118. https://doi.org/10.1016/S0140-6736(18)32427-9.

3 World Health Organization (2022). WHO European Regional Obesity Report 2022.

4 Qutteina, Y., De Backer, C., and Smits, T. (2019). Media food marketing and eating outcomes among pre-adolescents and adolescents: a systematic review and meta-analysis. *Obes. Rev.* 20: 1708–1719. https://doi.org/10.1111/obr.12929.

5 Balantekin, K.N., Anzman-Frasca, S., Francis, L.A. et al. (2020). Positive parenting approaches and their association with child eating and weight: a narrative review from infancy to adolescence. *Pediatr. Obes.* 15: e12722. https://doi.org/10.1111/ijpo.12722.

6 Maccoby, E.E. (1994). *The Role of Parents in the Socialization of Children: An Historical Overview*. Washington, DC: American Psychological Association https://doi.org/10.1037/10155-021.

7 Power, T.G., Sleddens, E.F.C., Berge, J. et al. (2013). Contemporary research on parenting: conceptual, methodological, and translational issues. *Child. Obes.* 9: S-87–S-94. https://doi.org/10.1089/chi.2013.0038.

8 van Strien, T., Beijers, R., Smeekens, S. et al. (2019). Parenting quality in infancy and emotional eating in adolescence: mediation through emotion suppression and alexithymia. *Appetite* 141: 104339. https://doi.org/10.1016/j.appet.2019.104339.

9 Favieri, F., Marini, A., and Casagrande, M. (2021). Emotional regulation and overeating behaviors in children and adolescents: a systematic review. *Behav. Sci. (Basel)* 11. https://doi.org/10.3390/bs11010011.

10 Kelly, N.R., Tanofsky-Kraff, M., Vannucci, A. et al. (2016). Emotion dysregulation and loss-of-control eating in children and adolescents. *Health Psychol.* 35: 1110–1119. https://doi.org/10.1037/hea0000389.

11 Christensen, K.A. (2019). Emotional feeding as interpersonal emotion regulation: a developmental risk factor for binge-eating behaviors. *Int. J. Eat. Disord.* 52: 515–519. https://doi.org/10.1002/eat.23044.

12 Boutelle, K.N., Braden, A., Knatz-Peck, S. et al. (2018). An open trial targeting emotional eating among adolescents with overweight or obesity. *Eat. Disord.* 26: 79–91. https://doi.org/10.1080/10640266.2018.1418252.

13 Shriver, L.H., Dollar, J.M., Calkins, S.D. et al. (2020). Emotional eating in adolescence: effects of emotion regulation, weight status and negative body image. *Nutrients* 13. https://doi.org/10.3390/nu13010079.

14 van Strien, T., Konttinen, H., Homberg, J.R. et al. (2016). Emotional eating as a mediator between depression and weight gain. *Appetite* 100: 216–224. https://doi.org/10.1016/j.appet.2016.02.034.

15 Kinasz, K.R., Ross, D.A., and Cooper, J.J. (2017). Eat to live or live to eat? The neurobiology of appetite regulation. *Biol. Psychiatry* 81: e73–e75. https://doi.org/10.1016/j.biopsych.2017.02.1177.

16 Li, Y.-J., Xie, X.-N., Lei, X. et al. (2020). Global prevalence of obesity, overweight and underweight in children, adolescents and adults with autism spectrum disorder, attention-deficit hyperactivity disorder: a systematic review and meta-analysis. *Obes. Rev.* 21: e13123. https://api.semanticscholar.org/CorpusID:221107506.

17 Hanć, T. and Cortese, S. (2018). Attention deficit/hyperactivity-disorder and obesity: a review and model of current hypotheses explaining their comorbidity. *Neurosci. Biobehav. Rev.* 92: 16.

18 Cortese, S. (2019). The association between ADHD and obesity: intriguing, progressively more investigated, but still puzzling. *Brain Sci.* 9: https://doi.org/10.3390/brainsci9100256.

19 Nigg, J.T., Johnstone, J.M., Musser, E.D. et al. (2016). Attention-deficit/hyperactivity disorder (ADHD) and being overweight/obesity: new data and meta-analysis. *Clin. Psychol. Rev.* 43: 67–79. https://doi.org/10.1016/j.cpr.2015.11.005.

20 Buro, A.W., Salinas-Miranda, A., Marshall, J. et al. (2022). Correlates of obesity in adolescents with and without autism spectrum disorder: the 2017–2018 national survey of children's health. *Disabil. Health J.* 15: 101221. https://doi.org/10.1016/j.dhjo.2021.101221.

21 Kamal Nor, N., Ghozali, A.H., and Ismail, J. (2019). Prevalence of overweight and obesity among children and adolescents with autism spectrum disorder and associated risk factors. *Front. Pediatr.* 7: 38. https://doi.org/10.3389/fped.2019.00038.

22 Cowling, I., Rashid, M.A., and Borrington, C. (1855). Obesity in young people with special educational needs – an audit of current practice. *BMJ Paediatr. Open* 2022: 6. https://api.semanticscholar.org/CorpusID:254808545.

23 Sammels, O., Karjalainen, L., Dahlgren, J. et al. (2022). Autism spectrum disorder and obesity in children: a systematic review and meta-analysis. *Obes. Facts* 15: 305–320. https://doi.org/10.1159/000523943.

24 Patel, B.P., Hamilton, J.K., Vien, S. et al. (2016). Pubertal status, pre-meal drink composition, and later meal timing interact in determining children's appetite and food intake. *Appl. Physiol. Nutr. Metab.* 41: 924–930. https://doi.org/10.1139/apnm-2016-0079.

25 Clark, T.D., Reichelt, A.C., Ghosh-Swaby, O. et al. (2022). Nutrition, anxiety and hormones. Why sex differences matter in the link between obesity and behavior. *Physiol. Behav.* 247: 113713. https://doi.org/10.1016/j.physbeh.2022.113713.

26 Klump, K.L., O'Connor, S.M., Hildebrandt, B.A. et al. (2016). Differential effects of estrogen and progesterone on genetic and environmental risk for emotional eating in women. *Clin. Psychol. Sci.* 4: 895–908. https://doi.org/10.1177/2167702616641637.

27 Luppino, F.S., de Wit, L.M., Bouvy, P.F. et al. (2010). Overweight, obesity, and depression: a systematic review and meta-analysis of longitudinal studies. *Arch. Gen. Psychiatry* 67: 220–229. https://doi.org/10.1001/archgenpsychiatry.2010.2.

28 Abou Abbas, L., Salameh, P., Nasser, W. et al. (2015). Obesity and symptoms of depression among adults in selected countries of the Middle East: a systematic review and meta-analysis. *Clin. Obes.* 5: 2–11. https://doi.org/10.1111/cob.12082.

29 Lamertz, C.M., Jacobi, C., Yassouridis, A. et al. (2002). Are obese adolescents and young adults at higher risk for mental disorders? A Community Survey. *Obes. Res.* 10: 1152–1160. https://doi.org/10.1038/oby.2002.156.

30 Quek, Y.-H., Tam, W.W.S., Zhang, M.W.B. et al. (2017). Exploring the association between childhood and adolescent obesity and depression: a meta-analysis. *Obes. Rev.* 18: 742–754. https://doi.org/10.1111/obr.12535.

31 Vilmann, L.S., Thisted, E., Baker, J.L. et al. (2012). Development of obesity and polycystic ovary syndrome in adolescents. *Horm. Res. Paediatr.* 78: 269–278. https://doi.org/10.1159/000345310.

32 Steegers-Theunissen, R.P.M., Wiegel, R.E., Jansen, P.W. et al. (2020). Polycystic ovary syndrome: a brain disorder characterized by eating problems originating during puberty and adolescence. *Int. J. Mol. Sci.* 21: https://doi.org/10.3390/ijms21218211.

33 Miller, W.R. and Rollnick, S. (2002). *Motivational Interviewing, Second Edition: Preparing People for Change.* New York: Guildford Press https://books.google.co.uk/books?id=r_CuyHwdz7EC.

34 Hooper, L., Puhl, R., Eisenberg, M.E. et al. (2022). How is weight teasing cross-sectionally and longitudinally associated with health behaviors and weight status among ethnically/racially and socioeconomically diverse young people? *Int. J. Behav. Nutr. Phys. Act.* 19: 1–15. https://doi.org/10.1186/s12966-022-01307-y.

35 Wang, S.B., Haynos, A.F., Wall, M.M. et al. (2019). Fifteen-year prevalence, trajectories, and predictors of body dissatisfaction from adolescence to middle adulthood. *Clin. Psychol. Sci.* 7: 1403–1415. https://doi.org/10.1177/2167702619859331.

36 Sequeira, G.M., Boyer, T., Coulter, R.W.S. et al. (2022). Healthcare experiences of gender diverse youth across clinical settings. *J. Pediatr.* 240: 251–255. https://doi.org/10.1016/j.jpeds.2021.08.089.

37 Williams, D.R., Chaves, E., Greenwood, N.E. et al. (2022). Care of gender diverse youth with obesity. *Curr. Obes. Rep.* 11: 215–226. https://doi.org/10.1007/s13679-022-00480-2.

38 Hastings, J., Geilhufe, B., Jaffe, J.M. et al. (2023). Creating inclusive, gender affirming clinical environments. In: *Reproduction in Transgender and Nonbinary Individuals: A Clinical Guide* (ed. M.B. Moravek and G. de Haan), 177–207. Cham: Springer International Publishing https://doi.org/10.1007/978-3-031-14933-7_13.

39 Goldenberg, T., Jadwin-Cakmak, L., Popoff, E. et al. (2019). Stigma, gender affirmation, and primary healthcare use among black transgender youth. *J. Adolesc. Health* 65: 483–490. https://doi.org/10.1016/j.jadohealth.2019.04.029.

40 Puhl, R.M., Himmelstein, M.S., and Watson, R.J. (2019). Weight-based victimization among sexual and gender minority adolescents: findings from a diverse national sample. *Pediatr. Obes.* 14: e12514. https://doi.org/10.1111/ijpo.12514.

41 Himmelstein, M.S., Puhl, R.M., and Watson, R.J. (2019). Weight-based victimization, eating behaviors, and weight-related health in sexual and gender minority adolescents. *Appetite* 141: 104321. https://doi.org/10.1016/j.appet.2019.104321.

42 Grammer, A.C., Byrne, M.E., Pearlman, A.T. et al. (2019). Overweight and obesity in sexual and gender minority adolescents: a systematic review. *Obes. Rev.* 20: 1350–1366. https://doi.org/10.1111/obr.12906.

43 Bishop, A., Overcash, F., McGuire, J. et al. (2020). Diet and physical activity behaviors among adolescent transgender students: school survey results. *J. Adolesc. Health* 66: 484–490. https://doi.org/10.1016/j.jadohealth.2019.10.026.

44 Johnson, K.C., LeBlanc, A.J., Deardorff, J. et al. (2020). Invalidation experiences among non-binary adolescents. *J. Sex Res.* 57: 222–233. https://doi.org/10.1080/00224499.2019.1608422.

45 Morales-Ghinaglia, N. and Fernandez-Mendoza, J. (2023). Sleep variability and regularity as contributors to obesity and cardiometabolic health in adolescence. *Obesity (Silver Spring)* 31: 597–614. https://doi.org/10.1002/oby.23667.

46 Chaput, J.-P. (2014). Sleep patterns, diet quality and energy balance. *Physiol. Behav.* 134: 86–91. https://doi.org/10.1016/j.physbeh.2013.09.006.

47 Kracht, C.L., Chaput, J.-P., Martin, C.K. et al. (2019). Associations of sleep with food cravings, diet, and obesity in adolescence. *Nutrients* 11: https://doi.org/10.3390/nu11122899.

48 Sunwoo, J.-S., Yang, K.I., Kim, J.H. et al. (2020). Sleep duration rather than sleep timing is associated with obesity in adolescents. *Sleep Med.* 68: 184–189. https://doi.org/10.1016/j.sleep.2019.12.014.

49 Sluggett, L., Wagner, S.L., and Harris, R.L. (2019). Sleep duration and obesity in children and adolescents. *Can. J. Diabetes* 43: 146–152. https://doi.org/10.1016/j.jcjd.2018.06.006.

50 Simon, S., Rahat, H., Carreau, A.-M. et al. (2020). Poor sleep is related to metabolic syndrome severity in adolescents with PCOS and obesity. *J. Clin. Endocrinol. Metab.* 105: e1827–e1834. https://doi.org/10.1210/clinem/dgz285.

51 Biddle, S., Whitehead, S., Odonovan, T. et al. (2005). Correlates of participation in physical activity for adolescent girls: a systematic review of recent literature. *J. Phys. Act. Health* 2: https://doi.org/10.1123/jpah.2.4.423.

52 Corr, M., McSharry, J., and Murtagh, E.M. (2019). Adolescent girls' perceptions of physical activity: a systematic review of qualitative studies. *Am. J. Health Promot.* 33: 806–819. https://doi.org/10.1177/0890117118818747.

53 Mahumud, R.A., Sahle, B.W., Owusu-Addo, E. et al. (2021). Association of dietary intake, physical activity, and sedentary behaviours with overweight and obesity among 282,213 adolescents in 89 low and middle income to high-income countries. *Int. J. Obes.* 45: 2404–2418. https://doi.org/10.1038/s41366-021-00908-0.

54 Biddle, S.J.H. and Asare, M. (2011). Physical activity and mental health in children and adolescents: a review of reviews. *Br. J. Sports Med.* 45: 886–895. https://doi.org/10.1136/bjsports-2011-090185.

55 World Health Organization (2023). Adolescent pregnancy: key facts. https://www.who.int/news-room/fact-sheets/detail/adolescent-pregnancy (accessed 18 February 2023).

56 World Health Organization (2020). Regional office for europe. Reducing Inequities in health across the life-course: early years, childhood and adolescence. https://iris.who.int/handle/10665/358239 (accessed 18 February 2023).

57 Yu, C.K.H., Teoh, T.G., and Robinson, S. (2006). Obesity in pregnancy. *BJOG* 113: 1117–1125. https://doi.org/10.1111/j.1471-0528.2006.00991.x.

58 Santos, S., Voerman, E., Amiano, P. et al. (2019). Impact of maternal body mass index and gestational weight gain on pregnancy complications: an individual participant data meta-analysis of European, North American and Australian cohorts. *BJOG* 126: 984–995. https://doi.org/10.1111/1471-0528.15661.

59 Berti, C., Elahi, S., Catalano, P. et al. (2022). Obesity, pregnancy and the social contract with today's adolescents. *Nutrients* 14: https://doi.org/10.3390/nu14173550.

60 Ameye, H. and Swinnen, J. (2019). Obesity, income and gender: the changing global relationship. *Global Food Secur.* 23: 267–281. https://doi.org/10.1016/j.gfs.2019.09.003.

61 Tod, E., Bromley, C., Millard, A.D. et al. (2017). Obesity in scotland: a persistent inequality. *Int. J. Equity Health* 16: 135. https://doi.org/10.1186/s12939-017-0599-6.

62 Moore Heslin, A., O'Donnell, A., Kehoe, L. et al. (2023). Adolescent overweight and obesity in Ireland-Trends and sociodemographic associations between 1990 and 2020. *Pediatr. Obes.* 18: e12988. https://doi.org/10.1111/ijpo.12988.

63 Lu, Y., Pearce, A., and Li, L. (2020). Distinct patterns of socio-economic disparities in child-to-adolescent BMI trajectories across UK ethnic groups: a prospective longitudinal study. *Pediatr. Obes.* 15: e12598. https://doi.org/10.1111/ijpo.12598.

64 Houtepen, L.C., Heron, J., Suderman, M.J. et al. (2020). Associations of adverse childhood experiences with educational attainment and adolescent health and the role of family and socioeconomic factors: a prospective cohort study in the UK. *PLoS Med.* 17: e1003031. https://doi.org/10.1371/journal.pmed.1003031.

65 Hemmingsson, E. (2018). Early childhood obesity risk factors: socioeconomic adversity, family dysfunction, offspring distress, and junk food self-medication. *Curr. Obes. Rep.* 7: 204–209. https://doi.org/10.1007/s13679-018-0310-2.

66 Adjei, N.K., Schlüter, D.K., Straatmann, V.S. et al. (2022). Impact of poverty and family adversity on adolescent health: a multi-trajectory analysis using the UK Millennium cohort study. *Lancet Reg. Heal. – Eur.* 13: 100279. https://doi.org/10.1016/j.lanepe.2021.100279.

67 Cicchetti, D., Rogosch, F.A., Gunnar, M.R. et al. (2010). The differential impacts of early physical and sexual abuse and internalizing problems on daytime cortisol rhythm in school-aged children. *Child Dev.* 81: 252–269. https://doi.org/10.1111/j.1467-8624.2009.01393.x.

68 Felitti, V.J., Anda, R.F., Nordenberg, D. et al. (1998). Relationship of childhood abuse and household dysfunction to many of the leading causes of death in adults. The Adverse Childhood Experiences (ACE) Study. *Am. J. Prev. Med.* 14: 245–258. https://doi.org/10.1016/s0749-3797(98)00017-8.

69 Hemmingsson, E. (2014). A new model of the role of psychological and emotional distress in promoting obesity: conceptual review with implications for treatment and prevention. *Obes. Rev.* 15: 769–779. https://doi.org/10.1111/obr.12197.

70 Michopoulos, V., Powers, A., Moore, C. et al. (2015). The mediating role of emotion dysregulation and depression on the relationship between childhood trauma exposure and emotional eating. *Appetite* 91: 129–136. https://doi.org/10.1016/j.appet.2015.03.036.

71 Gardner, R., Feely, A., Layte, R. et al. (2019). Adverse childhood experiences are associated with an increased risk of obesity in early adolescence: a population-based prospective cohort study. *Pediatr. Res.* 86: 522–528. https://doi.org/10.1038/s41390-019-0414-8.

72 Kim, Y., Lee, H., and Park, A. (2020). Adverse childhood experiences, economic hardship, and obesity: differences by gender. *Child Youth Serv. Rev.* 116: 105214. https://doi.org/10.1016/j.childyouth.2020.105214.

73 Davis, L., Barnes, A.J., Gross, A.C. et al. (2019). Adverse childhood experiences and weight status among adolescents. *J. Pediatr.* 204: 71–76. e1. https://doi.org/10.1016/j.jpeds.2018.08.071.

74 Waite, R. and Ryan, R. (2019). *Adverse Childhood Experiences: What Students and Health Professionals Need to Know*, 1e. New York: Routledge https://doi.org/10.4324/9780429261206 1e.

75 Bateman, J., Henderson, C., and Kezelman, C. (2014). Trauma-informed care and practice: towards a cultural shift in policy reform across mental health and human services in Australia, a national strategic direction.

76 Ko, S.J., Ford, J.D., Kassam-Adams, N. et al. (2008). Creating trauma-informed systems: child welfare, education, first responders, health care, juvenile justice. *Prof. Psychol. Res. Pract.* 39: 396–404. https://doi.org/10.1037/0735-7028.39.4.396.

77 Lee, E., Kourgiantakis, T., Lyons, O. et al. (2021). A trauma-informed approach in Canadian mental health policies: a systematic mapping review. *Health Policy (New York)* 125: 899–914. https://doi.org/10.1016/j.healthpol.2021.04.008.

78 Kuyken, W., Padesky, C.A., and Dudley, R. (2009). *Collaborative Case Conceptualization: Working Effectively with Clients in Cognitive-behavioral Therapy*. New York, NY: The Guilford Press.

79 Johnstone, L. and Dallos, R. (2013). *Formulation in Psychology and Psychotherapy: Making Sense of People's Problems*, 2e. London: Routledge.

13 Weight Management Considerations in Children Living with Special Educational Needs and Disability

Kiranjit Atwal and Laura Stewart

'To really understand that with a child and see what they are up against every day. It just puts you in their shoes and understand their subsequent behaviours'. [1]

Introduction

Excess weight can manifest more prominently in children and young people (CYP) with special educational needs and disabilities (SEND) compared to age-matched non-SEND peers [2]. CYP with SEND present with learning difficulties and/or physical disabilities which can impact their physical, intellectual and behavioural capacity [3]. Challenges that make attaining a healthy weight difficult in this population are many and may include low motor skills and subsequently low physical activity, selective eating habits and particular behaviours. Furthermore, lack of knowledge amongst families and low availability of tailored services are also key factors [4]. Successful weight management of CYP with SEND requires specialist knowledge and training to prevent inequalities in care. This will be explored in detail in this chapter.

Child and Adolescent Obesity: A Practical Approach to Clinical Weight Management,
First Edition. Edited by Laura Stewart.
© 2024 John Wiley & Sons Ltd. Published 2024 by John Wiley & Sons Ltd.

The term SEND will be used throughout this chapter. The scope of the term is broad and will include CYP with attention deficit hyperactivity disorder (ADHD), autism spectrum disorder (ASD), Down's syndrome, spina bifida and developmental delay which may co-exist [5].

Evidence in this population is scarce and of low quality due to poorly designed studies, and heterogenicity in definitions and reported outcomes. As such, there is not enough good quality data to support clinical guidelines and strong practice recommendations. Some of the evidence used in this chapter is broad and derived from children with a range of neurodevelopment (or neurodivergent) disorders and intellectual or learning disabilities. These terms may be otherwise defined within the original referenced papers used in this chapter, although underlying principles are similar. Caution should be exercised when generalising information from this chapter. Genetic (including, Prader-Willi, Barbet-Biedl, Cohen, Fragile X), neuromuscular and neurodegenerative disorders will not be specifically discussed but may be mentioned within the evidence used.

Prevalence

Globally, pooled prevalence estimates of overweight and obesity among those with SEND are 30% for children aged ≥4–11 years (of which 15% overweight and 13% obese) and 33% for adolescents aged ≥11–18 years (of which 18% overweight and 15% obese). These figures are based on data from a selection of countries in Europe, North and South America, the Middle East, East Asia and Australia [6]. Among children, the highest estimates were seen in North America versus the lowest in South Korea. Among adolescents, the highest estimates were seen in Australia, Turkey and North America, versus the lowest in France and South Korea [6]. However, the prevalence is likely underestimated [6].

Similar levels have also been reported in Northern Ireland among 33% of CYP [7]. Whereas Stewart et al. reported 36% prevalence of obesity from a survey of nine schools in Scotland, which was significantly higher in secondary schools (CYP aged 11–16) versus primary schools (children aged 5–11) [2].

Compared to non-SEND CYP, data has consistently shown that CYP with SEND demonstrate greater levels of obesity [8]. Data from British children aged five to eleven years found those with SEND exhibit persistent rates of obesity (11.2%) versus non-SEND children (8.2%) [9]. In contrast, recent data from low- and middle-income countries (such as Bangladesh and Kenya) suggests that obesity prevalence is much lower among SEND children than their healthy counterparts [10].

Challenges and Risk Factors

There are many potential challenges and risk factors that make CYP with SEND more susceptible to developing obesity. It is important to identify these in order to manage and prevent complications of obesity. The most common are discussed below.

Reduced Energy Requirements

It is likely CYP with Down's syndrome or other conditions may have low fat-free mass, low muscle tone and/or low activity levels as a result of their condition. As such, this may reduce energy requirements which can make CYP with SEND susceptible to weight gain. It is possible that estimations of energy using predictive equations risk overestimating energy needs in this group [11].

Limited Physical Ability

Recommendations for physical activity by the WHO for CYP from the age of five years suggest engagement in 60 minutes of moderate to vigorous intensity activity per day. It is also recommended that strengthening exercises be undertaken at least three times per day while sedentary time should be limited [12].

Some evidence suggests CYP with SEND fail to meet this target, have greater sedentary behaviours (including higher levels of screen time) and partake in lower intensity physical activity compared to non-SEND peers [7, 13, 14]. Furthermore, a negative correlation with physical activity has been identified with increasing age which may track into adulthood [15].

Reasons for low physical activity amongst CYP with SEND may be due to physical limitations (such as impaired motor skills or wheelchair use) or cognitive limitations (such as coordination or orientation) which may arise from underlying morbidity. This may fuel low self-confidence in exercise competency which may further reduce participation [16]. Screen time may also be used as a means to reduce or control challenging behaviours in a CYP which may subsequently decrease physical activity levels.

Selective Eating Habits

The prevalence of sensory-related food preferences in CYP with SEND is notably higher, particularly in those with ASD. This may give rise to 'selective' eaters based on the appearance, texture, temperature or smell of food. As such, consumption of energy-dense, nutrient-poor processed foods (such as fries) and refusal of fresh foods (such as fruits and vegetables) are common.

Consumption of fruits, vegetables and dairy in CYP with SEND are markedly lower compared to age-matched peers in some studies [7, 14]. Furthermore, in CYP with Down's syndrome, the consumption of fruits and vegetables may be challenging due to hindered mastication skills which can delay the introduction of certain foods and consistencies [17]. The CYP may also display challenging behaviours around food, snacks and meal times leading the parents and caregivers to avoid changing from high-energy foods and not introducing new foods.

Intellectual Ability and Behavioural Challenges

The level of intellectual ability in CYP with SEND may impact the day-to-day application of healthy lifestyle behaviours. For example, they may not understand the health risks of obesity or learn how to self-regulate their activity or food intake [18].

The presence of oppositional behaviours in CYP with ADHD (who typically have difficulty with hyperactive and impulsive behaviours) and ASD (who typically have disruptive or obsessive behaviours) may increase their risk of obesity if healthy lifestyle behaviours are resisted [19].

CYP with both ADHD and ASD can also experience problems with social communication which can impair their social participation. This may lead to greater sedentary behaviours or risk of inappropriate coping strategies, for example, the risk of comfort eating (although this has not been widely documented in the evidence) [18].

Condition-Specific Medication Side Effects

A number of commonly used medications for this group can have side effects that impact weight gain. Rapid weight gain and increased appetite have been observed in CYP with ASD-prescribed risperidone for severe behavioural challenges (irritability and aggression). However, links to metabolic syndrome have been demonstrated as possible side effects of risperidone use [20].

Methylphenidate and dexamphetamine prescribed in CYP with ADHD may decrease hyperactive and impulsive behaviours, but may also suppress appetite and slow growth [19].

While rarer, a small number of studies have highlighted the risk of weight gain from antipsychotic and antidepressant medications used in CYP with severe psychiatric and behavioural problems. This has been linked to medication side effects that include increased appetite [21].

Parenting Style

Parent or caregiver BMI and level of physical activity have been associated with the risk of obesity in CYP with SEND. Lack of awareness of healthy lifestyle behaviours amongst parents and caregivers, or use of overfeeding as a means of behaviour control or reward, may induce excess weight gain. Furthermore, overprotective behaviours in fear of injury or social isolation may create reluctance to involve children in physical activity [4, 14]. For discussions around challenging meal times behaviours and strategies to modify see Chapter 10.

Environment

It is known that those with SEND experience health inequalities and barriers to accessing adequate healthcare which places them at higher risk of disease. This may be related to stereotypes or stigma associated with their condition, which may lead to misunderstanding the abilities of CYP with SEND and the associated benefits or risks [22].

There are a lack of tailored and appropriately designed interventions available for CYP with SEND for physical activity and weight management programmes. Specific adaptions to meet the needs of individual CYP with SEND may also be lacking due to a lack of trained personnel. Where available, these may be inaccessible or associated with high expense which may pose a barrier for some families [4, 14].

Many healthcare services may not be able to meet the demand or needs of CYP with SEND due to a lack of funding or resources. There may also be a lack of social support services for CYP with SEND. For example, those transitioning into independent living settings may need guidance on purchasing food and meal planning, or support with transportation and taking part in physical activity sessions [4].

Growth Assessment

The experience of growth assessment for a CYP with SEND may be distressing, particularly if they have already experienced stigma as a result of their condition. Using simple language and explaining the purpose of weight measuring is important by focusing on its role in overall health promotion rather than determining the success of health alone.

It is important to involve the parent or caregiver in the process of growth assessment before any measurements are taken. It may be useful to discuss the CYP's learning ability and learning style with the parent or caregiver before having a conversation with the CYP. For example, visual (through the use of images and pictures such as those found on www.apictureofhealth.southwest.nhs.uk), auditory (through listening) or tactile (through activities and props). Some CYP may not fully understand what is happening and may appear to be non-cooperative. There will be some CYP with SEND who will not be able to engage themselves in the programme at all and all engagement will have to go through the parent/caregiver. Time and patience should be shown and advice on how best to help them understand should be discussed with their parent or caregiver.

Alternative Approaches to Weighing

Hoist weighing attachments are available for CYP who cannot use standing scales due to physical disabilities. Hoists allow the safe transfer of an individual from different positions, usually operated by an electrically powered sling on a metal frame. The hoist weighing attachment can be placed on the sling to record an individual's weight.

For wheelchair users, specific wheelchair scales with and without handrails may be available instead. These are robust for weighing while remaining seated in a wheelchair or, where appropriate, standing with assistance using handrails.

Segmental Growth Measures

It may be challenging to measure height if there are physical limitations or a CYP cannot weight bear. There is a lack of consensus in the literature between appropriate segmental measurements for linear growth such as knee-heel height or arm span in CYP. This is due to the risk of methodological error and low availability of reference standards [11].

Ulna length has been identified as a reliable segmental measure for linear growth by some healthcare professions, as a linear relationship has been found to exist with height in children aged 2–18 years. Estimated height can be extrapolated from ulna length measurements based on the Gauld equations [23, 24]:

2–6 Years

Males: 4.629*ulna + 1.340*age + 26.974
Females: 4.577*ulna + 1.343*age + 28.345

7–18 Years

Males: 4.605*ulna + 1.308*age + 28.003
Females: 4.459*ulna + 1.315*age + 31.485

Condition-Specific Growth Charts

Certain conditions can affect the rate at which a CYP grows. Where sufficient data is available, specific growth charts have been developed to monitor growth accurately in these populations. For example, in CYP with Down's syndrome who exhibit smaller stature and head circumference, specific growth charts are available from the UK-World Health Organization (WHO) or Centers for Disease Control and Prevention in North America [25, 26]. Some healthcare professionals argue that these are based on limited data sets, so monitoring on standard, country-specific or WHO growth charts may also be advised [27].

Components of Management

Many clinical guidelines in the management of CYP living with obesity do not address the specific needs of those living with SEND. Unfortunately, this conveys the lack of high-quality evidence, and thus inconsistencies in practice. Most general guidelines recommend a personalised, multi-component (diet, physical activity and behaviour change) approach [28–30]. The influence of limiting beliefs or stereotypes held on this population may limit the quality of care delivered. A person-centred, tailored approach is key for CYP living with SEND due to their varying degrees of presentation and need. Common features in multi-component interventions (diet, physical activity and behaviour change) from the best available evidence are discussed.

Aims of Management

Outcomes in CYP with SEND may be different from other CYP with excess weight due to the additional challenges and risk factors. A realistic weight goal may either aim for a slower rate of weight gain or weight maintenance to improve overall BMI. It is important that weight is not proposed as the sole marker of progress, but other outcomes such as reducing sedentary time are also considered.

Diet Concepts

Energy Deficit

Reducing energy intake may help to achieve weight loss in CYP with SEND, but has been rarely studied. In one study, energy reduction was based on 20–30% less energy than expected for weight in those with Down's syndrome and physical disabilities in CYP from as young as 2 years. Indirect calorimetry was also used, but its indication was poorly described, nor compared with aiming for a 20–30% energy deficit to establish any differences in weight loss outcomes [31]. A daily 250-calorie deficit was advised in another study on adolescents and young adults with SEND but was ultimately described as conservative, as the rate of weight loss was slower than expected [32].

Unfortunately, there is no consensus from the evidence on the efficacy or how to determine energy deficit. The impracticalities of indirect calorimetry in clinical practice would make the use of energy calculations a more favourable method of achieving an energy deficit. In practice, energy requirements may be no more than 75% of the estimated average requirements (EARs) for height age, but this may be too high even for some [11].

Simple Strategies

Following a nutritionally balanced diet based on MyPlate US and Eatwell plate UK, – see Chapter 7 which includes a reduction in energy with individualised goals for each client was the mainstay of most dietary interventions from the available evidence [31, 33, 34].

The use of the Traffic Light Diet is also popular amongst this group and has helped to promote weight loss in some studies [35, 36]. Categories of food are graded by energy content: red foods (those high in fat/calories), such as chips or cake, which are consumed once in a while; yellow foods (those lower in fat/calories), such as bread or pasta, which are consumed sometimes; and green foods (those lowest in fat/calories), such as fruits or vegetables, which are consumed frequently. However, individuals may have difficulty in differentiating and regulating intake of red and green foods [36]. See Chapter 6 for more details on the Traffic Light Diet.

A modified Traffic Light Diet with low-calorie meal replacements for 50% of energy intake has also been explored. However, no difference in weight loss was found between groups with and without the use of meal replacements [34]. Due to the sensory challenges common amongst this population, compliance with meal replacement may be difficult and may discourage the consumption of lower calorie, whole, fresh foods.

Physical Activity

In a systematic review of activity in CYP with SEND (predominantly with learning difficulties), several interventions were able to target weight loss, although there were mixed outcomes from multi-component interventions. These are recommended more strongly than physical activity interventions alone [37]. This may be due to the heterogenicity of the evidence with differences in duration (ranged from 2 to 9 months), frequency of activity (ranged from 1 to 3 times per week) and types of activity incorporated (ranged from aerobic, interval training, endurance training and/or walking), as well as types of disabilities studied.

Behaviour and Environment

Sensory-Food Integration

To overcome the sensory difficulties which can create food selectivity in the diet of CYP with SEND, the sequential oral sensory (SOS) approach was described in one study as part of the weight management intervention. Changes to the presentation of preferred food were made, for example, by shape, colour or texture, and food exposure was advanced through visual tolerance, interaction, smell, touch, taste, and eventually eating. In Gillette et al. oral sensory processing was observed during eating in the initial assessment with the multidisciplinary team [33]. Unfortunately, in much of the evidence, sensory-food integration was not discussed in detail.

Food chaining is a common method used to expand dietary variety in children with extreme food refusal. It is based upon building exposure to new foods linked to existing safe foods by similar characteristics (e.g., flavour, shape, consistency, and colour) [38]. This approach may help to contribute to a level of security for the CYP. Building trust and cooperation in the process for the CYP is important, as well as avoiding pressure from parents and caregivers, as this may negatively affect their CYP's eating experience.

Access

Stimulus control has been included as part of behavioural management in Gillette et al. but detail on how this was managed was not provided [33]. It is important to consider the parents and caregivers involved in looking after CYP with SEND may also need education on healthy lifestyle habits. This will help to minimise exposure to fast-food when taking a CYP out of home (by considering visiting places away from these outlets), or avoidance of food as a reward for good behaviour.

Routine

Meal and snack times can be a particularly challenging time for parents and caregivers, and often learnt eating behaviours are accepted to ease the situation. Recommending a consistent and planned approach to meal or snack patterns should be given, and these are discussed in depth in Chapter 6.

Considerations of Management

Family-Centred Interventions

Reliance on parents and caregivers for daily aspects of living may be particularly high if physical and/or cognitive deficits exist in CYP with SEND. As such, their involvement in healthy lifestyle change is essential. Consistently across the available evidence, family-centred interventions were implemented through involvement in education, goal setting and monitoring. Families received varied education on food shopping, physical activity, food monitoring, parenting skills and how to create environments to support change. Unfortunately, none of the studies identified or discussed which members of the family units were included, or the impact of intergenerational influence and blended families [34, 39, 40].

Social Learning Theory

Bandura's social learning theory underpinned the intervention in two studies on CYP with SEND (school and family-based interventions). This theory suggests that behaviour is learnt through observations and imitations of others within the social network (see Chapter 5). This can aid in effective lifestyle changes and decision-making. For example, health-related behaviours are learnt through instructors and teachers among peers and family members who act as collective role models in the CYP's environment (home and school) [39, 41]. Therefore, ensuring a whole family approach to changes to the family lifestyle is fundamental in supporting these changes in CYP with SEND.

Goal Setting

Goal setting forms a crucial part of weight management interventions and in CYP with SEND. It is important to understand the CYP's level of intellectual ability when co-building goals. The role of the parent or caregiver may aid or lead in goal setting accordingly. It is important not to assume that the CYP with SEND will be completely unable to input into co-building goals. While being aware that in some family situations, the parent or caregiver will be the one setting the goals. In one study, parents and caregivers were identified as 'agents of change' and in another study, one parent or caregiver from the family unit was identified to specifically facilitate change. They were involved in co-creating family-centred goals after identifying unhealthy household habits as well as aiding the CYP with SEND to meet their own goals [34, 39].

Communication

CYP with SEND may have learning difficulties which can make involvement in decision-making about their care challenging. Information should be presented at the level of a CYP's cognitive ability. Simple causes and effects of health behaviours should be discussed, and the delivery of messages through activities that could be enjoyed by the family unit may be beneficial. The use of complex language, being excluded by healthcare professionals and solely focused on the condition and/or its symptoms, may create barriers to care. A useful website is from the *mefirst organisation – Children and young people centred communication* (mefirst.org.uk). Using a person-centred approach to communicate will help a CYP to be understood, and feel involved in their care, and is less likely to create challenges for parents and caregivers which may improve the CYP's overall health outcomes [42, 43].

It is important to discuss the CYP's learning preference with the parent or caregiver and/or CYP to understand the best way to work with them. The CYP may have an education and healthcare plan in place which may already include some of this information.

If the CYP has a visual preference for learning, this helpful website (www.apictureofhealth.southwest.nhs.uk) has a useful image bank for explaining common concepts in healthcare. They may currently use a Picture Exchange Communication (PEC) system of communication [44] and images could be added to this. If the CYP has a listening preference using simple language is important, encouraging them to reflect back what they have understood might be helpful. If a CYP has a tactile learning preference, using photos of portion sizes or food models, live demonstrations and interactive games may aid learning [43].

Self-Monitoring

While self-monitoring is an important part of most weight management interventions, there is very little available evidence about adapting this for CYP with SEND. Few studies have involved the use of electronic technology (Fitbits and iPads) for monitoring diet and physical activity goals in CYP with SEND. Unfortunately, the ease at which technology was used by CYP with SEND was not explored [34, 35].

The use of such technology may be associated with a financial burden on healthcare budgets or for parents and caregivers. Furthermore, some technology may not provide enough detail on the type of data collected. For example, step counters may not pick up the intensity of activity. Simple self-monitoring charts can provide more simple yet useful feedback instead.

Group Versus One-to-One Interventions

The effectiveness between group and one-to-one weight management interventions for CYP living with SEND has not been compared. From the available evidence, dropouts from group interventions were high (approximately 50%) but similar to other reports of group weight management. Reasons for dropout were not explored but time commitment and accessibility may have been linked. Most of the CYP with SEND were from lower socioeconomic backgrounds; therefore, the financial burden of travel or the frequent time commitment (as much as weekly) may have created a barrier to participation [31, 33, 40, 41].

One study looked at the difference between intervention delivery modes (remote versus face-to-face). However, no difference in weight loss was observed amongst CYP with SEND. One of the limitations of this study was that participation was incentivised, which may have influenced compliance. Delivery mode, particularly remote, would be useful to further explore in light of recent healthcare demands following the COVID-19 pandemic. In a study on young adults, 80% attendance was recorded following weekly video chat with dietitians via a tablet for education on diet and physical activity [34]. While the benefits of remote delivery may help reduce financial burdens and save time for both the health service and the families, efficacy on weight and BMI outcomes need to be reliably proven [34]. It is important to note that each CYP with SEND may have individual communication styles which may include preference of face-to-face education.

Providing flexible interventions will allow for individual variation and a person-centred approach to treatment may be more helpful while no single intervention has been proven to be more effective than another.

Frequency of Contact

The frequency of contact in weight management interventions was highly variable in the evidence. In one intervention, this was as often as weekly for the first 6 months (24 sessions), then bi-weekly for the next 6 months (12 sessions), then either after 6 (2 sessions) or 12 months only (1 session). Those who received more frequent follow-ups lost further weight but after one year, all groups regained 1 kg [41]. Whereas other studies found weight loss with an average attendance of <5–6 sessions but did not provide follow-up after the initial intervention to understand the long-term impact [31, 33]. It is important to note that the funding available in studied programmes does not reflect what funding is available for staff time in most healthcare settings, which may limit the frequency of contact available.

Role of the Multidisciplinary Team

Interventions with specialist healthcare professionals have demonstrated successful outcomes through the person-centred management of obesity in CYP with SEND. From the evidence, these have included specialist nurses, paediatricians, dietitians, occupational therapists, psychologists and physical activity specialists (albeit the latter more uncommonly). While each had key roles, for example, occupational therapists conducted assessments on oral motor skills and oral sensory processing, their specific roles or interventions were inadequately described. In some cases, specialist healthcare professionals were present for the initial assessment, or entire duration of programmes, and all made recommendations. Unfortunately, in most of the available evidence, long-term involvement and roles of each specialist healthcare professional were not explored [31, 33, 34, 40].

Table 13.1 aims to propose a list of specific aspects and responsibilities of healthcare professionals in the weight management of CYP living with SEND:

Table 13.1 Aspects of weight management and responsibilities of healthcare professionals working CYP living with obesity and SEND.

Specific aspects of weight management	Responsible healthcare professional(s)
Diagnosis of underlying medical conditions (e.g. hypothyroidism)	Paediatrician/nurse
Poor knowledge on healthy eating	Dietitian
Reviewing medications that impact on appetite and weight gain	Paediatrician/pharmacist
Difficulties in managing challenging behaviours	Psychologist/nurse
Sensory processing issues impacting food choice, and meal time environment	Occupational therapist/ dietitian
Delayed oral motor skills impacting food choice	Speech and language therapist/dietitian
Poor motor skills and orientation to meet activity targets	Physical activity specialist
Low self-esteem/self-efficacy for implementing changes (behaviour change support)	Psychologist/nurse/dietitian
Social care standards not matched to child's requirements or additional support (carer needs)	Social care (social worker)
A young person transitioning into adult residential setting requiring assistance with food purchases and food preparation	Dietitian/social care (social worker)

This list is not exhaustive.

Summary

There are few specifically designed weight management interventions for CYP with SEND. What is highlighted is the importance of family involvement, follow-up, person-centred care and the multidisciplinary team as well as adaptations to address specific needs (for example, sensory food integration). Whilst it is difficult to recommend one approach over another, the evidence available does provide valuable insights into an area that has been inadequately researched. Future research should integrate the specific needs of CYP living with SEND and their families; take into account their intellectual and physical abilities and challenges; focus on the influence of peers, caregivers and the impact of the environment on health-related behaviours; and how to maintain a healthy weight long term.

WHAT DOES THIS MEAN IN PRACTICE?

- Interventions should be tailored and person-centred, aiming to involve the family unit to aid lifestyle changes.
- Healthcare professionals should work within a multidisciplinary setting and define their roles and responsibilities throughout the course of intervention.
- Communication style and preferences should be established with a CYP and/or their family in order to deliver effective care.
- Healthcare professionals should be aware of the additional risks and challenges in this population, and assess these in each individual.
- Specific strategies should be advised to address the needs of each CYP, and family-based goals should be established with both the CYP and family unit.
- Tailored resources should be used which may include visual aids, live demonstrations and where possible, access to physical activity specialists.
- Aspects of management such as self-monitoring and behavioural change are just as important and should be implemented with support from the parent or caregiver.
- Members of the weight management team should ensure that they undertake specific training so they have an understanding of behaviours and communication to support CYP with SEND.

References

1 Stewart, L. (2023). Personal communication: practitioner.
2 Stewart, L., Van de Ven, L., Katsarou, V. et al. (2009). High prevalence of obesity in ambulatory children and adolescents with intellectual disability. *J. Intellect. Disabil. Res.* 53 (10): 882–886.
3 GOV.UK. Children with special educational needs and disabilities (SEND). https://www.gov.uk/children-with-special-educational-needs (accessed 10 January 2023).
4 Bandini, L., Danielson, M., Esposito, L.E. et al. (2015). *Obesity in children with developmental and/or physical disabilities. Disabil. Health J.* 8 (3): 309–316.
5 Comer-HaGans, D., Weller, B.E., Story, C. et al. (2020). Developmental stages and estimated prevalence of coexisting mental health and neurodevelopmental conditions and service use in youth with intellectual disabilities, 2011–2012. *J. Intellect. Disabil. Res.* 64 (3): 185–196.
6 Maïano, C., Hue, O., AJS, M. et al. (2016). Prevalence of overweight and obesity among children and adolescents with intellectual disabilities: a systematic review and meta-analysis. *Obes. Rev.* 17 (7): 599–611.
7 Slevin, E., Truesdale-Kennedy, M., McConkey, R. et al. (2014). Obesity and overweight in intellectual and non-intellectually disabled children. *J. Intellect. Disabil. Res.* 58 (3): 211–220.
8 Krause, S., Ware, R., McPherson, L. et al. (2016). Obesity in adolescents with intellectual disability: prevalence and associated characteristics. *Obes. Res. Clin. Pract.* 10 (5): 520–530.
9 Emerson, E., Robertson, J., Baines, S. et al. (2016). Obesity in British children with and without intellectual disability: cohort study. *BMC Public Health* 16 (1): 644.
10 Savage, A. and Emerson, E. (2016). Overweight and obesity among children at risk of intellectual disability in 20 low and middle income countries. *J. Intellect. Disabil. Res.* 60 (11): 1128–1135.
11 Shaw, V. (2020). *Clinical Paediatric Dietetics*, 5e. Wiley-Blackwell.
12 WHO (2022). Physical activity. https://www.who.int/news-room/fact-sheets/detail/physical-activity (accessed 20 January 2023).
13 Einarsson, I., Ólafsson, Á., Hinriksdóttir, G. et al. (2015). Differences in physical activity among youth with and without intellectual disability. *Med. Sci. Sports Exerc.* 47 (2): 411–418.
14 Must, A., Curtin, C., Hubbard, K. et al. (2014). Obesity prevention for children with developmental disabilities. *Curr. Obes. Rep.* 3 (2): 156–170.
15 Phillips, A.C. and Holland, A.J. (2011). Assessment of objectively measured physical activity levels in individuals with intellectual disabilities with and without Down's syndrome. *PLoS One* 6 (12): e28618.
16 Hinckson, E.A. and Curtis, A. (2013). Measuring physical activity in children and youth living with intellectual disabilities: a systematic review. *Res. Dev. Disabil.* 34 (1): 72–86.

17 Cañizares-Prado, S., Molina-López, J., Moya, M.T. et al. (2022). Oral function and eating habit problems in people with Down syndrome. *Int. J. Environ. Res. Public Health* 19 (5): 2616.

18 Reinehr, T., Dobe, M., Winkel, K. et al. (2010). Obesity in disabled children and adolescents: an overlooked group of patients. *Dtsch. Arztebl. Int.* 107 (15): 268–275.

19 Sayal, K., Prasad, V., Daley, D. et al. (2018). ADHD in children and young people: prevalence, care pathways, and service provision. *Lancet Psychiatry* 5 (2): 175–186.

20 Scahill, L., Jeon, S., Boorin, S.J. et al. (2016). Weight gain and metabolic consequences of risperidone in young children with autism spectrum disorder. *J. Am. Acad. Child Adolesc. Psychiatry* 55 (5): 415–423.

21 Alonso-Pedrero, L., Bes-Rastrollo, M., and Marti, A. (2019). Effects of antidepressant and antipsychotic use on weight gain: a systematic review. *Obes. Rev.* 20 (12): 1680–1690.

22 Turner, S. (2014). Improving care for people with learning disabilities. *Nurs. Stand.* 29 (12): 53–59.

23 Gauld, L.M., Kappers, J., Carlin, J.B. et al. (2004). Height prediction from ulna length. *Dev. Med. Child Neurol.* 46 (7): 475–480.

24 Gauld, L., Keeling, L., Sly, P. et al. (2013). Predicting height from ulna length in 2–6 year olds. *Eur. Respir. J.* 42 (Suppl 57): P1265.

25 CDC (2020). Growth charts for children with Down syndrome. https://www.cdc.gov/ncbddd/birthdefects/downsyndrome/growth-charts.html#print (accessed 21 January 2023).

26 RCPCH (2023). UK-WHO growth charts – Down syndrome, 0–18 years. https://www.rcpch.ac.uk/resources/uk-who-growth-charts-down-syndrome-0-18-years (accessed 21 January 2023).

27 WHO (2006). The WHO Child Growth Standards. https://www.who.int/tools/child-growth-standards/standards (accessed 21 January 2023).

28 Ells, L.J., Rees, K., Brown, T. et al. (2018). Interventions for treating children and adolescents with overweight and obesity: an overview of Cochrane reviews. *Int. J. Obes.* 42 (11): 1823–1833.

29 NICE (2013). Weight management: lifestyle services for overweight or obese children and young people. https://www.nice.org.uk/guidance/ph47.

30 PHE (2017). A guide to commissioning and delivering tier 2 weight management services for children and their families. *Publ. Health Engl.* https://www.gov.uk/government/publications/child-weight-management-commission-and-provide-services (accessed 21 January 2023).

31 Pona, A.A., Dreyer Gillette, M.L., Odar Stough, C. et al. (2017). Long-term outcomes of a multidisciplinary weight management intervention for youth with disabilities. *Child. Obes.* 13 (6): 455–461.

32 Curtin, C., Bandini, L.G., Must, A. et al. (2013). Parent support improves weight loss in adolescents and young adults with Down syndrome. *J. Pediatr.* 163 (5): 1402–8.e1.

33 Gillette, M.L., Stough, C.O., Beck, A.R. et al. (2014). Outcomes of a weight management clinic for children with special needs. *J. Dev. Behav. Pediatr.* 35 (4): 266–273.

34 Ptomey, L.T., Washburn, R.A., Goetz, J.R. et al. (2021). Weight loss interventions for adolescents with intellectual disabilities: an RCT. *Pediatrics* 148 (3): e2021050261.

35 Ptomey, L.T., Sullivan, D.K., Lee, J. et al. (2015). The use of technology for delivering a weight loss program for adolescents with intellectual and developmental disabilities. *J. Acad. Nutr. Diet.* 115 (1): 112–118.

36 Weems, M., Truex, L., Scampini, R. et al. (2017). A novel weight-loss tool designed for adolescents with intellectual disabilities. *J. Acad. Nutr. Diet.* 117 (10): 1503–1508.

37 Conrad, E. and Knowlden, A.P. (2020). A systematic review of obesity interventions targeting anthropometric changes in youth with intellectual disabilities. *J. Intellect. Disabil.* 24 (3): 398–417.

38 Białek-Dratwa, A., Szymańska, D., Grajek, M. et al. (2022). ARFID-strategies for dietary management in children. *Nutrients* 14 (9): 1739.

39 Lee, R.L., Leung, C., Chen, H. et al. (2017). The impact of a school-based weight management program involving parents via mHealth for overweight and obese children and adolescents with intellectual disability: a randomized controlled trial. *Int. J. Environ. Res. Public Health* 14 (10): 1178.

40 Walker, M. and McPherson, A.C. (2020). Weight management services for an underserved population: a rapid review of the literature. *Disabil. Rehabil.* 42 (2): 274–282.

41 Bandini, L.G., Eliasziw, M., Dittrich, G.A. et al. (2021). A family-based weight loss randomized controlled trial for youth with intellectual disabilities. *Pediatr. Obes.* 16 (11): e12816.

42 HEE (2023). MeFirst: health education England. https://www.mefirst. org.uk/wp-content/uploads/2015/07/Me-first-PDSA-logbook.pdf (accessed 21 January 2023).

43 Grumstrup, B. and Demchak, M. (2017). *Obesity, nutrition, and physical activity for people with significant disabilities. Res. Advocacy Pract. Compl. Chron. Cond.* 36 (1): 13–28.

44 Bondy, A. and Frost, L. (2001). The picture exchange communication system. *Behav. Modif.* 25 (5): 725–744.

14 Obesity, Safeguarding and Child Protection

Rhian Augustus, Shelley Easter, and Laura Stewart

'I think for me one of the most challenging things is probably the fact that the complexity of the families, certainly in my experience, that we see'. [1]

Introduction

While childhood obesity is a ubiquitous public health issue, there remains ambiguity and debate as to whether it should be considered a child protection concern. This chapter aims to explore the role of services, safeguarding and child protection processes when there are concerns regarding a CYP living with obesity. It will explore the role of professionals working directly with the CYP and their family as well as the impact that an intervention may have on the identified risks and outcomes. Along with exploring the experiences of families and practitioners that support families where weight has been identified as a risk.

Why Do We Need to Know About Safeguarding?

It is vital to know about safeguarding, as everybody who works with CYP has a responsibility to ensure that CYP are kept safe and protected from harm. This includes knowing how to identify concerns and when to respond to them. All health and social care professionals working with CYP have an obligation to be aware of their local policies, procedures and the pathway for escalating safeguarding issues. On an organisational level, there are legal obligations that must be followed, and these may be different depending on your sector and country. These may vary between countries and regions and even vary between the four countries of the UK. In the context of working with families in a health setting within weight management, it is important to have knowledge of the legislation that provides guidance for working with CYP and families and an understanding of individual and organisational responsibilities. In the United Kingdom, a good resource for getting an understanding of safeguarding is the NSPCC website (Keeping children safe|NSPCC), as well as government websites directly, for example:

- **Scotland Getting it right for every child (GIRFEC)** – gov.scot (www.gov.scot)
- **England** – Working together to safeguard children – GOV.UK (www.gov.uk)
- **Australia** – Child protection Overview – Australian Institute of Health and Welfare (aihw.gov.au)

Through this chapter, UK policy and procedures around safeguarding and child protection will be explored as examples of practice.

Does This Mean that All CYP Living with Obesity Need a Safeguarding Response?

No, not all, but it is important to ask this question when working with families in which there are complications and health implications. How would you know when a CYP is at risk of significant harm and how do you escalate concerns and consider thresholds for services?

In order to be able to act to protect CYP, having an understanding of how to assess a CYP's holistic needs, identify harm, manage concerns and know what to do to support families in a proportionate manner is essential. Understanding why a CYP is living with obesity, if this is caused by neglect or is an indicator that it is as a response to traumatic events needs to be considered alongside an understanding of trauma, neglect and indicators of harm. Working together statutory guidance states that *'Neglect is characterised by the absence of a relationship of care between the parent/carer and the child and the failure of the parent/carer to prioritise the needs of their child. It can occur at any stage of childhood including the teenage years'* [2].

What Do We Mean by Safeguarding?

In the United Kingdom, safeguarding is the action that is taken to promote the welfare of CYP and protect them from harm. This includes protecting CYP from abuse and maltreatment, preventing harm to CYP's health or development, ensuring CYP grow up with the provision of safe and effective care, taking action to enable all children and young people to have the best outcomes [3].

In order to achieve this, the organisation that you work for may set up safeguarding training, policies and procedures. These will make sure that everyone knows how to recognise and respond to concerns, regularly review safeguarding arrangements, keep up to date with best practice and the latest guidance. Along with formal training, this may be achieved through supervision meetings with practitioners that are adept at working with families where there are safeguarding needs.

'Safeguarding children' is an umbrella term for any of the actions that achieve the above aims. It could be described as a spectrum with varying degrees of statutory and non-statutory involvement depending on the needs of a CYP and the level of harm and risk. It may involve one agency, universal services that any CYP can access right through to specialist services that need referrals and thresholds met. A CYP may need support through early help and voluntary community services, children's social care including CYP in need, child protection interventions and CYP in care. Knowledge of these services and processes are often supported by specialist safeguarding practitioners within teams and organisations but sometimes as the only professional working with a family it is important to understand these processes. Threshold documents produced by children's social care front door/multi-agency safeguarding hubs (MASH) teams or local safeguarding children boards are designed to help practitioners working with CYP identify when additional support may help CYP achieve their potential and keep them safe from harm.

Child protection is a term often referred to when discussing safeguarding; in the United Kingdom, it is a statutory process that is part of safeguarding CYP. It involves working to protect CYP that are or likely to suffer significant harm. This chapter will explore roles within this statutory process; as previously stated, these may be referred to in different terms.

What Does This Mean When Working with CYP and Families?

When a CYP is referred for support, it is important to get a thorough understanding of their needs. This requires practitioners to be skilled in communication and be able to analyse and verify the information being shared. Having a holistic approach may be tricky if you have a very specific role with a CYP, but, as discussed, all professionals are responsible for safeguarding. Having your own child centred plans in order to support families should be the first step to consider, unless there are any immediate safeguarding concerns that need addressing. This may be a clinic letter or more structured meal plans or change goals and tasks provided in an accessible format to families. These plans may change over time as rapport and relationships develop as well as changing needs. Having a child-centred approach can help to keep the CYP central to the intervention and focus on what the impact of any concern or risk is on the CYP. In serious case reviews, which will be discussed later in this chapter, there is a learning point identified where CYP's voice and needs are overlooked when working with adults who also have their own needs that required support.

In Scotland, all professionals working with CYP use the same system for holistically identified positives and challenges for the CYP, with the CYP being in the centre of the assessment. This is worked through under the *Getting it right for every child policy* [4]. The professional/s works through the eight aspects of the acronym *SHANARRI* to make an assessment:

> '**Safe** – *growing up in an environment where a child or young person feels secure, nurtured, listened to and enabled to develop to their full potential. This includes freedom from abuse or neglect.*
>
> **Healthy** – *having the highest attainable standards of physical and mental health, access to suitable healthcare, and support in learning to make healthy and safe choices.*
>
> **Achieving** – *being supported and guided in learning and in the development of skills, confidence and self-esteem, at home, in school and in the community.*
>
> **Nurtured** – *growing, developing and being cared for in an environment which provides the physical and emotional security, compassion and warmth necessary for healthy growth and to develop resilience and a positive identity.*
>
> **Active** – *having opportunities to take part in activities such as play, recreation and sport, which contribute to healthy growth and development, at home, in school and in the community.*
>
> **Respected** – *being involved in and having their voices heard in decisions that affect their life, with support where appropriate.*
>
> **Responsible** – *having opportunities and encouragement to play active and responsible roles at home, in school and in the community, and where necessary, having appropriate guidance and supervision.*
>
> **Included** – *having help to overcome inequalities and being accepted as part of their family, school and community'* [4].

When considering what needs to happen for a CYP and constructing a plan, it is important that what is being put in place has a meaningful impact, for example if a goal that is identified is that a CYP attends all appointments, explain why this is important and what outcomes are being focused on, and what meeting that goal looks like. Breaking down larger longer-term goals in a way that is a positive, collaborative and achievable adopts a solution-focused approach that could be used in interventions with families [5, 6].

As part of an MDT, effective sharing of information and joint working can ensure that a clear and meaningful plan can be made with families. This may set out what needs to happen and who needs to take action. Being able to share this with families and professionals within the team and the wider network is useful as it can be a way to track what changes have been made and if they are being maintained. Considering accessibility of information is also important in terms of how CYP and their families are able to receive and understand information. Consider if verbal or written information needs to be translated or provided in a format that enables it to be understood by CYP and their families.

Being Able to Recognise Signs of Harm in CYP

Working Together defines neglect as *'The persistent failure to meet a child's basic physical and/or psychological needs, likely to result in the serious impairment of the child's health or development'*. [2]

In your role with CYP you may want to reflect upon how the risks and impact of living with obesity and its complications are assessed and perceived. When there are indicators of neglect, are these being perceived as a purely medical issue by other agencies? If parents are not able to make changes for their CYP despite support being provided, there needs to be time and a process where the professional/s can objectively consider how a CYP's health is being impacted in the short and longer term. Reflection and discussions then need to take place on how this is acted upon whilst still being proportionate and managing expectations.

It is important to distinguish between fact and opinion when responding to and recording concerns. Being specific about what the risks are to a CYP and what impact this has, e.g. what health complications are directly related to a CYP's weight and what this means in the short and longer terms for them. Deciding whether what has been heard as part of the session reflects what is being seen in terms of the CYP in question.

When making judgements and forming a professional opinion consider the following questions:

- What would you expect to see in your role supporting a CYP that would help you understand what is happening for a CYP?
- As part of a weight management team how do you get an understanding of when a CYP's needs are not being met?

Reflecting upon what you know about a CYP, as well as linking up with other professionals who know the CYP would be helpful in understanding why things are difficult. It is easy sometimes for our concerns to be heightened based on unknown information or missing parts of the puzzle.

Signs that may need further support or investigation may be:

- **A pattern of missed appointments** – both for your service and within the wider team or network.
- Attending appointments but not being able to implement changes in terms of food or activity levels suggested by the team, despite these being child centred and delivered in an accessible way for families.
- Weight escalating despite insistence that plans are being followed, this includes consideration of disguised compliance.
- **Health complications** – deterioration or worsening impact of weight.
- **Escalating concerns within the community** – e.g. isolation, not attending school or activities, deteriorating mental health, ongoing needs within family networks which means the child is not prioritised.
- Disclosures of trauma or abuse.
- Worries in terms of families not being able to change long-standing routines or behaviours without more specialist support.

CYP living with disabilities are more likely to suffer abuse and neglect than non-disabled CYP, as well as suffering multiple abuses [7]. Signs of abuse or neglect are often missed or mistaken as being part of their condition. Your professional responsibility may be to ensure that you have adequate training regarding the needs of CYP living with disabilities. Consider if any members of your MDT have specialist skills or resources to empower CYP to communicate their needs. CYP living with disabilities are more likely to rely on their parents or carers to meet their needs, which may make it difficult when trying to talk about their experiences.

An ongoing part of any intervention should be to assess the parenting capacity around any CYP that is referred to your service. Working with parents to support them to meet their child's needs is crucial. Building a relationship with the parent and the CYP will help you to understand parental behaviour and their ability to meet their child's needs and maintain change.

Adverse Childhood Experiences and Trauma Informed Practice

Adverse childhood experiences (ACEs) are not only important to understand the CYP that you support but also in terms of parents and carers as this may impact on parenting styles (see Chapter 10), capacity and their work with you. Research indicates that exposure to ACEs is linked to increased multiple difficulties including mental health difficulties, poor physical health and risky behaviours [8]. Understanding what a family has been through will help inform your assessment as well as the intervention. Your work may not be directly with parents in terms of their own needs but identifying how you can support or signpost parents to address or mitigate the longer-term effects will support whole families. Early intervention and prevention can support people from experiencing the effects of ACEs into adulthood.

This understanding as well as adopting a trauma-informed approach can provide a framework for your intervention that may provide a more holistic understanding of the CYP's needs. Trauma-informed care is an approach that aims to provide care on an individual and organisational level that seeks to understand and be responsive to the impact of trauma on the CYP [9]. The principles of trauma-informed practice will support young people and their families who face stigma within services not to be re-traumatised and to try to address their barriers to engaging. Substance Abuse and Mental Health Services Administration (SAMHSA)'s trauma-informed approach is based on a set of four assumptions (4 'R's') – Realize, Recognize, Respond and Resist Re-Traumatization and six key principles: safety – physical and psychological; trustworthiness and transparency; peer support; collaboration and mutuality; empowerment, voice and choice; and cultural, historical and gender acknowledgement [9]. All of which provide a framework for practice that provides not only a better experience for CYP but also a better understanding of need and therefore more appropriate intervention.

Safeguarding Stages

Early Help/Intervention

What to do when things are not improving or more help is needed? When there are worries that a family may need more support than one agency can provide, a step to consider is whether a network of support can be established around a CYP. With parental consent, establishing communication with professionals who already work with the family is good practice to form a 'team around the child' (different areas or countries may refer to this process in different terms). As a group of professionals, multi-agency communication is key so that both risks and safety for a CYP is accurately understood. When considering a plan that is accessible, it is useful to include the family to identify barriers to engagement and change, what may help to improve the situation and the responsibilities and actions of everyone around the CYP. Remember putting plans in place that are unrealistic may be setting families up to fail and negatively impact engagement. It is therefore essential that the plans that you create are both realistic and achievable for the family. As you get to know a family or CYP, other services may be identified to refer to in order to address some of their outstanding needs. This may be for support around state benefits or finances, activities, domestic abuse, organisations that support cultural needs or advocacy services. Some of the more useful support will be in the community and include interventions such as parenting groups or classes that can support a network to be able to look at boundary setting, which would inevitably link in with and improve engagement with the work of the MDT. Two such evidence-based courses are Triple P (Positive Parenting Programmes – Triple P Implementation|Official Corporate site) and The Incredible Years (Evidence-Based Early Intervention Programs|Incredible Years). Both of these programmes are delivered internationally.

Identifying spaces and activities that CYP can attend where they feel supported and not stigmatised may be helpful if a CYP or their family consent to further referrals. If CYP have more complex needs it might be extremely difficult to find services that could meet their needs. Within the United Kingdom, most local authorities must have databases that list services that can be accessed and what level of support they provide, within England this is called the 'local offer' [10]. Alternatively, establishing professional networks within local communities where resources and knowledge are shared will create an understanding of what support is available to families. This also may be as part of a community of practice with others in your field or sector.

There should also be consideration of when CYP and families are achieving goals:

- What provision is there for things to be maintained when your involvement has finished?
- What safety planning or steps should be taken if things are not maintained?
- Can there be a re-referral into your service or would there be other services that you refer onto that would know what to do should they become concerned?

You should share plans with community services such as the GP and school and give parents or carers clear guidance when approaching transition out of your service.

Social Care Involvement

When CYP have complex needs or concerns are escalating, children's social care teams may become involved. In England, this may be voluntarily under a child in need plan or with more statutory processes such as under Child Protection plan or as a child in care. As part of an MDT, involvement in these processes is vital and can be mandatory, so it is good to understand your role. Within different countries these processes may differ and it is important to understand the local structure of statutory services.

If a CYP on your caseload is open to the local authority or statutory services, it is good practice to be involved in the process. When involvement is voluntary, this would be with the permission of parents or carers. Being able to contribute to assessments, meetings and plans is essential if concerns include their health and associated complications. Often basic information is not passed on through networks and in isolation may not seem of great importance, but may help build up a more complete picture of what is happening for a CYP. Serious case reviews have identified that working in silos and a lack of inter-agency communication as a consistent feature where there has been serious harm to a CYP. Even ensuring that basic steps such as sharing meeting minutes and plans is vital as it sets out expectations both of families and the network around the CYP.

Some information that you may be asked to share is a summary of engagement with yourself or your team:

- What concerns do you have for the CYP?
- What positives/strengths/safety do you see around the CYP?
- What dietary changes or plans have been made with a family and what impact have these had?
- What is the engagement with the wider MDT and are treatment plans being followed, e.g. medication adherence?

Sharing any goals or outcomes that you have been reviewing and what impact any service or support has had if any.

CYP who are vulnerable due to their complex needs may also have involvement with social care due to their need for longer-term support or care, e.g. disabled children's teams. This may provide opportunity for you to discuss what can be put in place for a CYP where there is an established care network, or explore whether there would be funding through a direct payment or any entitled benefits (e.g. the UK's Disability Living Allowance) for a CYP to access a service or activity that needs additional support or staffing.

Plans with CYP and families should always be regularly reviewed and decisions made over whether there needs to be an escalation or step down should be based on risk and safety, using evidence-based professional judgement. You should be asked to contribute to multi-agency discussions when things are not progressing and when there needs to be more statutory involvement, such as a child protection plan. When considering outcomes, risks, safety and what changes need to happen for a CYP, you need to be critical of that information and what you are measuring. For example, you may be asked for weights/BMIs and patterns of change. It is important that these are viewed as part of a wider picture of the CYP and what is happening around them. In terms of your role, evidencing what these numbers mean and relating them to any impact on the CYP. A CYP's weight/BMI alone should never be seen as a reason for safeguarding or child protection.

When CYP are subject to more statutory involvement, you may be asked to share information regarding risk, and depending on the situation this may be as part of a child protection conference or a core group. In theory, this involvement should not change your work with the family and your input should continue as discussed throughout. Again, this is a continuation of the need for good inter-agency communication and co-operation as anyone supporting a CYP should be involved in this process. During this process, plans that are put in place for CYP are regularly reviewed, and risk and safety outcomes are monitored. Being fully aware about these plans increases safety for CYP.

Safeguarding leads or teams within organisations should be able to support with your work with families. This may be in formal supervision sessions as well as ongoing training and awareness of current research and practice with families. There may also be times when there are professional differences of opinion regarding families. In the United Kingdom, local authorities have escalation procedures in place if there are worries such as a referral is not progressed or concerns about the safety and well-being of a CYP are escalating despite support in place, and these are unable to be resolved as part of a multi-agency group. This may occur when professionals have little understanding of the impact of living with obesity and when it is overly medicalised.

As part of your role, you may be asked for your professional opinion when information needs to be shared in a legal forum or for legal purposes. This again needs to be something that you are supported with by your organisation and manager in terms of their formal processes.

Children in Care

When CYP are taken into the care of the local authority, this is an inevitably traumatic experience for the CYP and their families. This along with trauma and abuse may have led to the need to be in a different home environment and may have implications on eating patterns and coping strategies of a CYP, i.e. non-hunger eating, binge eating. This change in environment will be an opportunity for change and for families to be able to work with professionals to address what has led up to this point and reduce any identified risks. When CYP are taken into care, continuing the input by the MDT is important in order to ensure that the new environment is supportive. To help facilitate this, professionals should share any existing plans with any new carers. Providing continuity of care and maintaining relationships is vital as there are often changes in staff and teams that come with becoming a child in care. Being in a new home environment may provide the opportunity for change that a CYP and family may need, especially when the goal is reunification with parents and carers.

As with the previous intervention, it is important that communication is maintained with social care teams and for there to be input into the plans and reviews that are held for the CYP.

There also needs to be a consideration regarding what the new home environment looks like and what changes need to be made with the new carers to meet the CYP's needs in terms of your involvement. If this is a foster placement, foster carers should be invited alongside parents, if safe to do so, to attend appointments. If it is a residential home, then establish a key contact so that care plans can be put in place that take into consideration what the CYP has experienced and what was being put in place prior to the transition into care.

Legislation and Guidance

In England, the legal framework for professionals working with CYP and families are The Children Acts of 1989 [11] and 2004 [12] and statutory guidance working together to safeguard children [2]. They set out specific duties, section 17 of the Children Act 1989 puts a duty on the local authority *'to provide services to children in need in their area'* and section 47 of the same Act requires *'local authorities to undertake enquiries if they believe a child has suffered or is likely to suffer significant harm'* [10]. As a professional working alongside CYP, it would be your contribution, either as an individual or as part of the wider MDT's professional opinion that would form an understanding of whether a child is likely to suffer or has suffered significant harm. This would be evidenced with regards to health and the impact of any complications.

Despite there being government guidance with regards to approaches to address childhood obesity [13, 14], there is very little statutory guidance for social service involvement. Only a few local safeguarding boards [15, 16] adopt clear guidance with regards to weight management. This guidance is based on a framework proposed by Viner et al. to support professionals to make decisions and understand child protection concerns [17]. However, this framework is not universally adopted, known to professionals or evaluated in terms of its usefulness or application in practice [18].

Despite not being official guidance, following a serious case review of a death of a child [19], the authors suggest that based on the Viner et al. [17] framework that a safeguarding referral should be made where:

- *'There is a lack of acceptance of professional advice*
- *There is a consistent failure on the part of a parent/carer to change lifestyle and to address the concerns regarding a pattern of behaviour which is underpinning the obesity*
- *Complete parental/carer inability to take responsibility for their part in the problem and willingness to create change; the extreme end of this is where the parent/carer blames the child completely for the problem and is negative and denigrating of the CYP*
- *Lack of attendance of appointments, poor compliance with treatment regimens and when there is a lack of engagement/hostility towards professionals*
- *The existence of co-morbidities such as asthma, sleep apnoea, joint problems, weight related injuries (sprains, breaks etc.), incontinence, skin conditions and diabetes*
- *The CYP outcomes are compromised by the obesity, e.g., social presentation/interaction with peers/educational attainment*
- *Concerns are escalating over time'* [19].

What Research Tells Us

As discussed throughout this book, childhood obesity is acknowledged as a public health concern and has significant impact on the health, development and emotional well-being of CYP both in the short and long terms [2, 20, 21]. Despite the recognised risks and increasing numbers of CYP who are living with overweight or obesity, particularly in deprived areas [22], opinion is divided on whether a CYP's weight should be a child protection concern and limited research into the role of children's services intervention adds to this lack of good quality evidence.

In 2020, Peter Nelson et al. [18] undertook qualitative research into childhood obesity and child protection in one local authority in Northern England. The authors interviewed professionals working in health, social care and education to gather views on child protection and obesity. Their findings suggest threshold judgements are inconsistent, and this may be limiting access and acceptance of services. These decisions are also being made on personal judgement rather than medical evidence. Participants were divided on whether childhood obesity should be a child protection concern, but it was more likely to be viewed as such when families did not engage with services that were being offered. They comment that the current data on the number of CYP coming into the care of the local authority is hard to find, and there is little research on the outcomes of these interventions [18].

A Swedish study investigated the impact of placing CYP with 'severe obesity' into foster placement debated the balance between a parent's rights and a CYP's right to health [23]. They found a positive effect on health, social and psychological outcomes for the CYP that were placed in foster care; however, they also found varying effects when CYP were placed in kinship placements. Case studies from a medical perspective also document the impact of placing a CYP in foster care due to their weight which resulted in a reduction in BMI [24]. This research echoes that weight was not the only concern for the CYP and the need for all other avenues of support to be explored to justify removal from birth family.

Serious Case Reviews

Recent serious case reviews in the United Kingdom have reflected common themes as learning points for professionals that work with CYP where there are concerns about excess weight. In this section, three case reviews are briefly summarised.

The 2022 learning review report from Hampshire of a child named Grace showed the difficulties when a child has complex needs, including a medical diagnosis that was presented as an explanation for the signs of neglect. Following a period of weight loss during an inpatient stay, there was little evidence of sustained change by parents once at home and her weight increased to the point where she needed urgent medical intervention. There was a pattern of missed appointments and parents not being compliant with medical treatments and equipment provided for complications related to her excess weight. This resulted in the local authority obtaining an interim care order due to the risk of harm to her [25].

A 2018 serious case review was conducted following the death of Child F1 in Manchester from a heart condition that was exacerbated by them living with severe obesity. Child F1 was seen by many professionals in different services over many years. The review suggests learning for professionals in terms of understanding childhood obesity, understanding and responding to signs of neglect, difficult conversations with parents about weight and adopting a psycho-social approach to assessing needs [19].

A 2018 serious case review of a child named R in Lothian, Scotland, noted they were living with severe obesity when they were admitted to hospital due to complications of severe nutritional deficiency. Although child R had severe obesity, they were not under the care of a weight management team. The case review report noted that family interrelationships needed to be considered, especially where these had led to developmentally inappropriate and/or inconsistent interactions with the child's needs, that severe obesity is not easily managed, while it can significantly negatively affect the CYP's long term health, the possible rare complications of obesity are not understood or always recognised by professionals. There should be medical and/or dietetic oversight in cases of severe obesity. With MDT and multi-agency, SMART planning is important. Progress should be monitored and child safeguarding procedures used when necessary to help improve the well-being and protection of CYP [26].

Learning from the Serious Case Reviews

As is common in serious case reviews, it was highlighted that agencies need to work together, information being shared and concerns being escalated appropriately. Multi-agency communication to share concerns of issues such as missed appointments, engagement and compliance could have been improved in many of the reviews.

There were concerns that not enough is known about childhood obesity, its complications and understanding when it indicates neglect, significant risk of harm and when it should be escalated.

The over medicalisation of a CYP's needs may lead to issues of neglect and safeguarding concerns being missed as this limited the psycho-social assessment of the CYP's needs being considered.

Being able to effectively assess parenting capacity, prioritising the needs of the parents instead of ensuring that the plans were child centred and meaningful. This included identifying and addressing disguised compliance and parent's ability to maintain change.

A lack of professional curiosity and not challenging the narrative of parents and carers meant that a CYP's voice was not heard and acted upon.

In summary, many of the learning points from these serious case reviews echoes learning from most case reviews in terms of the need for the CYP 's voice and needs to be understood and prioritised. When thinking about your role with families, implementing learning and recommendations, consider how as an individual or MDT you can ensure that systems are set up in a way that guarantees information is understood and shared at an appropriate time. Consider what best practice looks like in your role, how your approach and work with CYP can ensure that you are prioritising their voice and needs.

WHAT DOES THIS MEAN FOR PRACTICE?

Safeguarding is everyone's responsibility and you should be familiar with your local polices as well as legal frameworks and statutory guidance.

Adopt a holistic and child-centred approach when implementing changes.

Develop an understanding of ACEs and adopt a trauma-informed approach to support CYP to understand their needs and improve outcomes.

Use professional curiosity and skills to gather and critically analyse information within the context and knowledge of your role.

A CYP's weight alone should not trigger a safeguarding response. Identifying it as an indicator of neglect and understanding parenting capacity to meet a CYP's needs may need further support to make and sustain changes.

Multiagency communication is crucial when there are concerns and to build a more holistic picture.

Opportunities for reflection within the MDT and with supervisors adept at safeguarding can be a useful tool.

References

1 Stewart, L. (2021). Personal communication: practitioner.
2 Department for Education (DfE) (2018). Working together to safeguard children. A guide to inter-agency working to safeguard and promote the welfare of children. [London]: Department for Education (DfE). https:// assets.publishing.service.gov.uk/media/5fd0a8e78fa8f54d5d6555f9/ Working_together_to_safeguard_children_inter_agency_guidance.pdf (accessed 18 September 2023).
3 NSPCC learning (2023). Safeguarding children and child protection. https://learning.nspcc.org.uk/safeguarding-child-protection (accessed 18 September 2023).
4 The Scottish Government (2012). The Scottish Government. A guide to getting it right for every child. http://www.scotland.gov.uk/ gettingitright/publications%0Ahttp://www.scotland.gov.uk/ Resource/0042/00423979.pdf (accessed 05 October 2023).
5 Shennan, G. (2014). *Solution-Focused Practice: Effective Communication to Facilitate Change*. Basingstoke, Hampshire: Palgrave Macmillan.
6 NSPCC Learning (2015). Solution-focused practice toolkit: helping professionals use the approach when working with children and young people. nspcc.org.uk.
7 Jones, L., Bellis, M., Wood, S. et al. (2012). Prevalence and risk of violence against children with disabilities: a systematic review and meta-analysis of observational studies. *Lancet* 380: 899–907. https://doi.org/10.1016/ S0140-6736(12)60692-8.

8 Schroeder, K., Schuler, B.R., Kobulsky, J.M. et al. (2021). The association between adverse childhood experiences and childhood obesity: a systematic review. *Obes. Rev.* 22 (7): e13204.

9 Substance Abuse and Mental Health Services Administration (2014). *SAMHSA's Concept of Trauma and Guidance for a Trauma-Informed Approach. HHS Publication No. (SMA) 14-4884.* Substance Abuse and Mental Health Services Administration: Rockville, MD.

10 Department for Education (DfE) (2018). Local offer guidance Guidance for local authorities. https://assets.publishing.service.gov.uk/government/uploads/system/uploads/attachment_data/file/683703/Local_offer_guidance_final.pdf (accessed 12 September 2023).

11 Children Act 1989, c41. https://www.legislation.gov.uk/ukpga/1989/41/contents (accessed 14 September 2023).

12 Children Act 2004, c31. http://www.legislation.gov.uk/ukpga/2004/31/contents (accessed 14 September 2023).

13 Childhood obesity; a plan for action https://assets.publishing.attachment_data service.gov.uk/government/uploads/system/uploads/attachment_data/file/546588/Childhood_obesity_2016__2__acc.pdf (accessed 19 October 2023).

14 Welsh Government. Healthy weight: Healthy Wales (2021). Weight management pathway 2021: children, young people and families. https://www.gov.wales/sites/default/files/publications/2021-06/all-wales-weight-management-pathway-2021-children-young-people-and-families.pdf (accessed 12 October 2023).

15 Norfolk Safeguarding Children partnership (2023). Safeguarding response to obesity when neglect is an issue. https://norfolklscp.org.uk/about/policies-procedures/children-in-specific-circumstances/523-safeguarding-response-to-obesity-when-neglect-is-an-issue (accessed 19 September 2023).

16 Suffold safeguarding board; safeguarding response to obesity when neglect is an issue. https://static1.squarespace.com/static/62ea37b2f412d231ae2c2f35/t/63932262165f001c6717f5ae/1670586979810/Safeguarding+Response+to+Obesity+when+Neglect+is+an+Issue.pdf.

17 Viner, R.M., Roche, E., Maguire, S.A., and Nicholls, D.E. (2010). When does childhood obesity become a child protection issue? *BMJ* 341 (7769): 375–377.

18 Nelson, P., Bissell, P., Homer, C. et al. (2021). Is childhood obesity a child protection concern? *Br. J. Soc. Work* 51 (8): 2944–2963. https://doi.org/10.1093/bjsw/bcaa100.

19 Wiffin, J. and Morgan, A. (2018). Child F1: serious case review. Manchester safeguarding children board. https://www.manchestersafeguardingpartnershiplearning.co.uk/learning-from-serious-case-reviews-scr-f1-course-2473 (accessed 15 September 2023).

20 Guh, D.P., Zhang, W., Bansback, N. et al. (2009). The incidence of co-morbidities related to obesity and overweight: a systematic review and meta-analysis. *BMC Public Health* 25 (9): 88. https://doi.org/10.1186/1471-2458-9-88. PMID: 19320986; PMCID: PMC2667420.

21 Reilly, J.J., Methven, E., McDowell, Z.C. et al. (2003). Health consequences of obesity. *Arch. Dis. Child.* 88 (9): 748–752. https://doi.org/10.1136/adc.88.9.748.

22 NHS England, Lifestyles team. (2023). National child measurement programme, England, 2022/23 school year. https://digital.nhs.uk/data-and-information/publications/statistical/national-child-measurement-programme/2022-23-school-year (accessed 15 September 2023).

23 Regber, S., Dahlgren, J., and Janson, S. (2018). Neglected children with severe obesity have a right to health: is foster home an alternative? A qualitative study. *Child Abuse Negl.* 83: 106–119. https://doi.org/10.1016/j.chiabu.2018.07.006.

24 Williams, G.M.G., Bredow, M., and Barton, J. (2014). Can foster care ever be justified for weight management? *Arch. Dis. Child.* 99: 297–299.

25 Hampshire safeguarding children partnership; learning review report Grace. https://www.hampshirescp.org.uk/wp-content/uploads/2022/11/Hampshire-Learning-Summary-Grace-with-Board-Response-Published-1-February-2022.pdf (accessed 15 September 2023).

26 Logie, L. and East Lothian and Midlothian Public Protection Committee (2019). Significant case review Child R: executive summary. East Lothian and Midlothian: East Lothian and Midlothian Public Protection Committee. https://blogs.glowscotland.org.uk/glowblogs/public/fvpp/uploads/sites/9924/2019/08/14154343/SCR-East-and-Midlothian-Child-R-February-2019.pdf (accessed 14 September 2023).

About the Editor

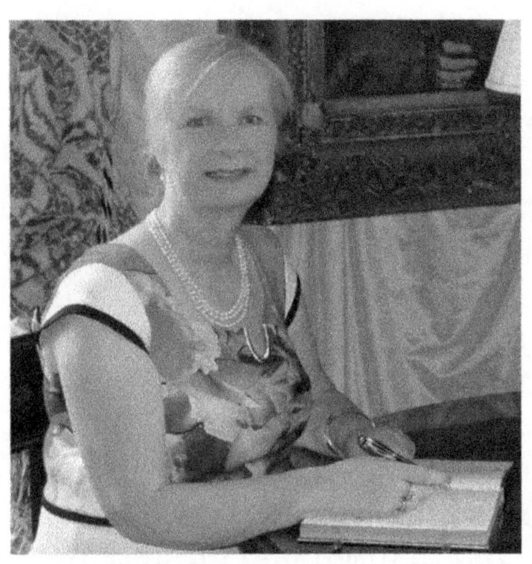

Dr Laura Stewart, PhD, BSc, BA, RD
Lead Consultant, Appletree Healthy Lifestyle Consultancy, Scotland, UK

Dr Laura Stewart is an award-winning registered dietitian who worked in the NHS for close to 38 years. For the last 20 or so of those years, she has specialised in the management of childhood obesity – as a practitioner, manager and researcher. Her PhD, from the University of Glasgow, was on the dietetic management of childhood obesity. Laura spent two years as a Professional Adviser to the Scottish Government on implementing their Type 2 Diabetes Prevention Framework. She now runs her own business, Appletree Healthy Lifestyle Consultancy, specialising in training the workforce on childhood obesity and supporting weight management services.

Laura's awards include the British Dietetics Association's Ibex Award for commitment to the dietetic profession and the 2006 Elizabeth Washington Award for best dietetic published educational article. Laura was a member of the 2003 Scottish Intercollegiate (SIGN) working group on the management of childhood obesity (SIGN 69) and the 2010 working group on the management of obesity (SIGN 115) guidelines. She recently led the writing team that developed five e-learning modules on childhood obesity for NHS England, with the writing team winning the BDA's 2024 Elizabeth Washington Award for this piece of work.

Notes on Contributors

Dr Jenny Gillespie, PhD, BSc (Hons) Health Sciences with Nutrition, BSc (Hons) Nutrition & Dietetics, RD
A registered dietitian with over 17 years of experience working in the NHS in clinical, public health and research roles, with an interest in the management and prevention of childhood obesity. Between 2019 and 2023 supported the co-production of a local child healthy weight strategy, lead the implementation and local evaluation of Scottish Government 'early adopter' Whole Systems Approach (utilising Public Health England's Whole Systems Approach to Obesity Guide). Awarded a PhD from the University of Strathclyde, Glasgow, in 2022 with a research study that focused on the translation and feasibility testing of a pre-school, childhood obesity prevention intervention. Between 2008 and 2020 delivered evidence-based individualised and group-based Childhood Weight Management Interventions alongside children, young people, families and communities in Scotland.

A published author in a number of peer-reviewed journals, textbooks and reports.

Dr Julie Lanigan, RD, PhD, FBDA
Julie Lanigan is a clinical dietitian specialising in paediatric weight management, an academic researcher and lecturer with more than 25 years of experience in paediatric nutrition and dietetics. She is currently investigating the effects of early nutrition on long-term health of children at UCL Institute of Child Health, London. Julie is the founding director of Trim Tots Community Interest Company set up by UCLB to develop evidence-based interventions for the prevention and treatment of childhood obesity. She co-created and directs the Planet Munch Healthy Lifestyle Programme for pre-school children.

Child and Adolescent Obesity: A Practical Approach to Clinical Weight Management,
First Edition. Edited by Laura Stewart.
© 2024 John Wiley & Sons Ltd. Published 2024 by John Wiley & Sons Ltd.

Julie has supervised many PhD students on a diverse range of projects including clinical projects, multi-centre infant feeding trials and studies involving cultural adaptations and feasibility assessments of the Planet Munch Healthy Lifestyle Intervention for prevention of obesity in pre-school children in the United Kingdom and overseas.

Julie has published widely, including more than 60 original research articles and several book chapters. She is a regular invited speaker at national and international conferences and lectures on childhood nutrition at UCL and the University of Plymouth. Most recently Julie has joined the editorial board of the *Journal of Human Nutrition and Dietetics* as Associate Editor.

She is also a programme lead for the paediatric dietetics master's programme at the University of Plymouth.

Dr Clare Q Neilson, MA (Hons), DClinPsychol, BABCP
Clare is an experienced Consultant Clinical Psychologist who has worked in the NHS in Scotland for over 25 years. During much of her career she has worked as part of an MDT within a weight management team, and it is within this team that she has worked with children, young people and their families who have sought professional help to manage their weight. Having worked in this life-span way, Clare is passionate about the need for early intervention and ultimately the prevention of the long-term conditions associated with overweight and obesity. Having had the privilege to work with many families, children and young people, Clare is heartened to see in first hand the developments there have been in the delivery of trauma-informed practice because so often people's relationship with food has evolved as a reaction to early life trauma. The complexity around weight management is also something that Clare is keen to educate others' professionals about, and the way professionals speak to people living with overweight and obesity can further compound those early life trauma experiences, serving to perpetuate that relationship with food further.

Shelley Easter, BSc, RD
Shelley is an experienced dietitian in the field of childhood weight management. She has worked for Bristol Royal Hospital for Children for 18 years within the CoCO team (Care of Childhood Obesity), and this is now one of the NHSE CEW (Complications from Excess Weight) sites. Shelley has helped produce NHSE's e-learning training package 'Complications from Excess Weight in children and young people' and the British Dietetic Association's Paediatric group's resource package called the obesity tool kit. Shelley has also contributed to a number of published papers including the British Dietetic Association's Obesity Specialist Group dietetic obesity management interventions in children and young people: review and clinical application.

Judith Cruikshank, MBA, MA

Judith is an independent behaviour consultant who has been working with children with language and developmental delays since 2004. After leaving secondary education, she held a number of administrative roles in the private sector, the NHS and a higher education institution and gained her Master of Business Administration in 2000. With a view to changing career, she returned to university as a mature student in 2003 and studied a degree in psychology. During these studies, she took up a part-time position as a tutor on a home-based applied behaviour analysis programme and experienced the joy of seeing the achievements individuals made. Deciding this was an area she wanted to further pursue and assist children to reach their full potential she continued her studies in this field and became Scotland's first board certified behaviour analyst in 2009 and set up ABA Scotland in the same year.

She is currently continuing her work as an independent behaviour consultant providing home-based educational programmes across Scotland for preschool-aged children with developmental and communication delays. She provides parent training on strategies to assist their child to develop preschool skills in areas such as communication, play skills and self-help skills. To maintain her skills Judith attends workshops, conferences and seminars on current research and development within the field of applied behaviour analysis and verbal behaviour.

Kiranjit Atwal, RD

Kiranjit is an experienced paediatric dietitian with over 10 years of experience. Kiranjit has a strong passion for supporting families and children living with obesity, which has formed an integral part of her career in many forms. Kiranjit has contributed to the field through the development of resources for the British Dietetic Association and training for NHS England/Health Education England. Furthermore, Kiranjit has managed and developed healthy lifestyle programmes including Trim Tots and KickStart, the latter of which went onto to win the Westminster Active Award in 2014.

Rhian Augustus

Rhian is a social worker in the UK.

Index

Please note that page numbers referring to Figures are followed by the letter '*f*', while references to Tables are followed by the letter '*t*'. 'CYP' stands for 'children and young people'.